PREFACE

The purpose of this book is to help users assess their knowledge of some of the main concepts of audiology. It can be used by students taking audiology classes or comprehensive examinations or preparing for major tests such as state and national examinations required of both audiologists and speech-language pathologists for certification and state licensure.

Often students of audiology are not certain that they have learned the important materials from notes and textbooks. This book is designed to allow readers to test their knowledge by completing specific exercises based on facts and concepts that were learned from such sources as textbooks and lectures. There is evidence that learning and reinforcement of learning increase with writing, and so the user of this book is encouraged to fill in the appropriate spaces provided and then check the answers at the end of each unit. Wherever possible, higher levels of learning are stressed, including application, synthesis, and generalization.

Part I contains twenty units whose contents can be used with almost any audiology textbook. Each unit deals with a specific area of audiology and attempts to utilize a variety of approaches to facilitate learning. In addition, fifteen case studies are provided in Part II, each of which presents a patient's history and some audiometric and other data. On the basis of this information, the reader should be able to determine the type and degree of hearing loss, discern the probable cause of the disorder, explain why those conclusions were reached, and make recommendations for proper case management.

Readers may use any primary sourcebook or class notes to fill in any missing information. It is important for readers to diagnose their own knowledge deficiencies and correct them in the best and most expeditious way possible in order to enjoy the good feeling that the material has been learned and retained. The following section will provide further direction on the best ways to use this book.

HOW TO USE THIS BOOK

Part I: Review Units

This book was designed to provide little in the way of new information but to assist readers in their efforts to monitor their own grasp of different aspects of audiology. When necessary, the reader should return to a textbook or lecture notes for needed information. Therefore, the study of each subject should be completed before a given unit in this book is attempted. The purpose here is to augment, rather than substitute for, previous learning. The reader is expected to take the responsibility, with the aid of this book, for determining which areas require further review and study. If an incorrect answer remains misunderstood, the reader should return to a primary source for further explanation.

The table of contents lists the twenty units reviewed in this book and the fifteen case studies. Each unit should be approached in the same way, although the order in which the units are studied may be determined by the needs and wishes of the reader. Some may be omitted entirely if that is desired. The following approaches are suggested:

1. Read the background material.
2. Read the stated objectives for each unit.

3. Complete the matching section to review the vocabulary of each subject.
4. Complete the outline for each unit. Write the letter that corresponds to a term from the right-hand column next to the appropriate number in the outline.

The completed outline will provide a framework for review. The purpose of the outline is to help you organize particular subjects. It is more than a mere matching exercise. You are forced to consider choices carefully because sometimes several items in the "Select From" column may be inserted into the outline in more than one place. Of course, if you wish to see the subject organization of a particular unit without doing the outline, the answers may simply be copied from the back of the unit. The decision on whether to approach the outline with this strategy is left to the individual.

5. In those units with activities, write the answers directly in the book. This may entail additional matching, labeling, drawing graphs, or other activities.
6. Circle the correct answer to each multiple-choice question—do not just assume that you will remember it.
7. On a separate sheet of paper write out the definition of each term in the vocabulary lists and compare it to the definitions given in a textbook glossary or a dictionary of audiological terminology. If you are uncertain of the definitions of some of the terms in the matching exercise, you should review a primary text. The greater your working vocabulary, the better your chances for a successful understanding of audiology.
8. When you have completed a unit, check your answers against those at the end of each unit.

For many people, completing the units in this book is preparation for an examination. Once a unit has been completed satisfactorily, or the reader recognizes weak points or corrects misconceptions, the sense of preparation can provide the sort of peace of mind that is always desirable before an examination. Those readers who do not do as well on a unit as they had hoped should be able to identify areas of deficiency quickly so that reviewing and learning the material can proceed logically.

Part II: Case Studies

Each theoretical case study is three pages long and represents a clinical diagnostic entity. Read the history statement on the first page. Then look at the audiogram, tympanogram, and other audiometric data on the second page. After you have reached your conclusions, fill in the appropriate spaces on the first page. Write down the probable etiology (cause) of each hearing disorder. Under "Case Management," write how you would handle the case, to whom a referral might be made, what might be said or written in a report, and so forth. Then write the reasons for your decisions. After this is done, check what you have written against the answers.

If more information is required to make a diagnosis, read the appropriate chapter in a textbook. The conditions described in the case studies are listed in alphabetical order in the table of contents, but they are not referred to by page because it is your task to identify the particular disorder from the information provided. Listing the disorders by page numbers would reveal the correct diagnosis ahead of time. You may observe that in the case studies more theoretical test results are presented than are usually obtained in routine practice. This is to illustrate the theoretical findings if all these tests had been performed.

ELEMENTS OF AUDIOLOGY

A Learning Aid with Case Studies

FREDERICK N. MARTIN

The University of Texas at Austin

JOHN GREER CLARK

University of Cincinnati and *Clark Audiology, LLC*

Boston   New York   San Francisco
Mexico City   Montreal   Toronto   London   Madrid   Munich   Paris
Hong Kong   Singapore   Tokyo   Cape Town   Sydney

To Dr. Mark Ross, my close friend and colleague for fifty years, for his many contributions to people with hearing loss and to the profession of audiology.

FNM

To Canon Kitty: friend, advisor, mentor, and mother for over fifty years.

JGC

Executive Editor and Publisher: Stephen D. Dragin
Production Editor: Gregory Erb
Editorial Production Service: Walsh & Associates, Inc.
Electronic Composition and Interior Design: Publishers' Design and Production Services, Inc.

For related titles and support materials, visit our online catalog at www.ablongman.com.

Between the time the website information is gathered and then published, it is not unusual for some sites to have closed. Also, the transcription of URLs can result in typographical errors. The publisher would appreciate notification where these errors occur so that they may be corrected in subsequent editions.

ISBN 0-205-48696-7   Complete Library of Congress Cataloging-in-Publication data can be provided upon request.

Printed in the United States of America

10 9 8 7 6 5 4 3 2 1   RRD-VA 10 09 08 07 06

CONTENTS

DISORDERS DESCRIBED IN
CASE STUDIES

Acoustic neuroma
Brainstem lesion
Central auditory lesion
Collapsed ear canal
Congenital hearing loss
Ménière disease
Meningitis
Noise-induced hearing loss
Nonorganic hearing loss—bilateral
Nonorganic hearing loss—unilateral
Obscure auditory dysfunction
Otitis media
Otosclerosis
Presbycusis
Serous effusion

AUDIOLOGICAL MANAGEMENT

BACKGROUND

In 1988 audiologists formed a new association, ". . . of, by and for audiologists," known as the American Academy of Audiology (AAA). In the years that have followed, the profession has made significant strides toward autonomy of practice in the management of hearing and balance disorders. All of the diagnostic audiological information gathered on a patient is useless unless it translates into some form of constructive action that helps the patient to communicate. Certainly it is in this arena that audiologists find their greatest autonomy.

Diagnosis of the type and degree of a patient's hearing loss is an essential beginning to audiological (re)habilitation. When possible, medical or surgical reversal of hearing loss is preferable. When this is impossible, or when the treatment does not result in sufficient functional hearing, steps must be taken to improve the patient's communicative abilities by utilizing residual hearing. For proper management, audiologists must become sophisticated in the intricacies of history taking, skilled in the provision of diagnostic assessments, adept in the development of a supportive relationship with their patients (or families), and both collegial and professional in their interactions with others who may be involved in the treatment of their patients.

Research has demonstrated the profound impact that hearing loss may have, not only for children and their families, but also for adults with hearing loss and their significant others. Large-scale studies have documented that untreated hearing loss increases levels of depression, anxiety, anger, and frustration. The increases in functional and psychosocial impact secondary to pediatric- and adult-onset hearing loss have been shown to decrease significantly through the use of corrective amplification and a strong course of audiological management.

High on the list of measures to be considered in audiological management is the selection, verification, and validation of proper hearing aids when indicated, as well as the provision of needed orientation to the use, care, and maintenance of amplification. Although drill work with adults in speechreading or discrimination of sounds is still practiced, it is considered by many clinicians not to be the most effectual means of audiological management for most patients. Many clinicians today construct the hearing-loss management they provide around hearing-handicap scales, completed by the patient, to help to judge the kinds of communicative difficulties that are experienced. Individual or group hearing management may include instruction designed to enhance the recognition of and intervention for those variables within the environment or poor speaker or listener habits that impede successful communication.

When working with children, audiologists must muster every resource at their disposal, including interactions with caregivers and other professionals, in designing approaches that will maximize the human potential in every child with a hearing loss. Audiologists find that working with the pediatric population brings them in close collegial contact with speech-language pathologists and classroom teachers. It is the pediatric audiologist's responsibility to understand the laws that have been implemented to ensure the best education for children with disabilities and to be able to help guide parents through the maze of options for the education of their children.

Underlying the success of the hearing-care services provided to adult patients as well as children and their caregivers is an effective approach to the counseling provided. Audiologists should be aware of the impact their words carry when what has sometimes become routine to audiologists is heard for the first time by those they are treating. Audiologists must learn to listen attentively to ensure that they recognize the frequently masked emotional underpinnings of the statements and questions patients and families ask. And audiologists need to recognize the stress that families with hearing loss live with, and that expressions of frustration and anger are rarely a reflection on the audiologist, but rather a reflection of the difficult circumstances that any disability brings in its wake. Although a good portion of the audiologist's education concentrates on the diagnosis of auditory disorders, practicing audiologists soon discover that sensitive audiological management should always be the culmination of their efforts.

OBJECTIVES

1. You should know and understand the terms in the matching exercise.

2. You should be able to fill in the outline, selecting items from the list provided.

3. You should try to understand some of the feelings of many patients with hearing disabilities so that these may be dealt with more efficiently.

4. You should understand the basic principles of speechreading training.

5. You should understand the basic principles of auditory training.

6. You should understand the basic principles of patient counseling.

7. You should be able to answer the multiple-choice questions.

8. You should know and understand the terms in the vocabulary list and be able to describe or define each term.

MATCHING

Match the term from the column on the right with its definition.

Definition

1. ___ A class of closely related speech sounds

2. ___ The production of speech as it appears on the lips

3. ___ The reeducation of individuals who have lost their hearing in listening for specific auditory cues

4. ___ The use of facial cues to determine the words of a speaker

5. ___ The recording of all background information related to a hearing loss

6. ___ A ringing or other sound heard in the ears or the head

7. ___ Any part of a word that conveys meaning

8. ___ Group instruction to help surmount variables within the environment, or poor speaker or listener habits, that impede successful communication

9. ___ Therapy to maintain clear articulation when auditory feedback of speech production has been decreased by postlinguistic hearing loss

Term

a. Auditory retraining

b. Hearing therapy

c. History taking

d. Morpheme

e. Phoneme

f. Speech conservation

g. Speechreading

h. Visime

i. Tinnitus

OUTLINE

Audiological (Re)habilitation	*Select From*
Speechreading	**A.** Adjustment to hearing aids
1. ___	**B.** Analytical methods
2. ___	**C.** Combined with residual hearing
3. ___	**D.** Communication guidelines
4. ___	**E.** Coping strategies
	F. Group counseling
Auditory Training	**G.** Individual counseling
5. ___	**H.** Hearing aid orientation
6. ___	**I.** Social strategies
7. ___	**J.** Word recognition in noise
8. ___	**K.** Word recognition in quiet
	L. Synthetic methods
Counseling	**M.** Support groups
9. ___	**N.** Tolerance for loud sounds
10. ___	**O.** Visible phonemes
11. ___	
12. ___	
13. ___	
14. ___	
15. ___	

MULTIPLE CHOICE

1. Important to a course in auditory training is the teaching of
   a. discrimination among speech sounds
   b. discrimination of speech sounds from nonspeech sounds
   c. discrimination of sound from silence
   d. all of the above

2. Speech detection implies
  a. sensing whether a sound is present
  b. the nature of a particular sound
  c. discrimination among speech sounds
  d. all of the above

3. Identification of speech sounds by a patient may be indicated by
  a. repeating the sound
  b. pointing to a picture or item
  c. writing down what was heard
  d. all of the above

4. *Auditory retraining* is a term used to denote that
  a. the hearing loss was adventitious
  b. the hearing loss was congenital
  c. the hearing loss was inherited
  d. all of the above

5. Audiological rehabilitation is usually most difficult for a patient with a moderate hearing loss that is
  a. conductive
  b. mixed
  c. sensorineural
  d. unilateral

6. The term *habilitation* is usually used when describing work with
  a. very young children
  b. teenagers
  c. adults
  d. the elderly

7. Aural rehabilitation often involves teaching adults to
  a. utilize contextual cues in speech
  b. make reasonable guesses
  c. predict language patterns
  d. all of the above

8. The least difficult listening situation for the new hearing aid wearer is
  a. understanding in quiet places
  b. understanding in noisy places
  c. understanding rapid speakers
  d. understanding unusual vocabulary

9. Patients wearing hearing aids can learn to improve the signal-to-noise ratio when listening in a noisy place by
   a. raising the volume of the hearing aids
   b. moving closer to the speaker
   c. asking the speaker to talk louder
   d. b and c

10. A basic assumption that may be made when hearing aids are provided to a small child is that
    a. speech will be clearer
    b. speech will be louder
    c. speech will be louder and clearer
    d. visual cues are unnecessary

11. A first step in an audiological habilitation program with a small child is sound
    a. repetition
    b. awareness
    c. discrimination
    d. production

12. Although there is some disagreement, most clinicians believe that audiological habilitation should include
    a. visual cues alone
    b. auditory cues alone
    c. visual and auditory cues combined
    d. none of the above

13. Of the more than 40 phonemes used in English discourse, approximately ____ are clearly visible
    a. 90 percent
    b. 20 percent
    c. 33 percent
    d. 5 percent

14. Most difficult to speechread are
    a. vowels
    b. consonants
    c. words in context
    d. sentences

15. Many audiologists believe that speechreading ability
    a. can be taught equally to all patients
    b. is a talent possessed more by some people than by others

     c. is unimportant if properly fitted hearing aids are used

     d. is easily learned

16. The ability to speechread is affected by

     a. the available light

     b. distance from the speaker

     c. rate of the speech

     d. all of the above

17. It is important to teach visual memory when teaching speechreading because

     a. speech is usually not repeated

     b. speech is rapid

     c. speech sounds, once seen, cannot be reviewed

     d. all of the above

18. SHHH is an acronym for

     a. Silence Here for Hard of Hearing

     b. Still Have Hearing Handicap

     c. Self Help for Hard of Hearing People

     d. Should Holler for Hard of Hearing

VOCABULARY

analytical speechreading methods	morpheme
auditory training	phoneme
group aural rehabilitation	psycholinguistics
hearing aid orientation	speechreading
individual aural rehabilitation	synthetic speechreading methods
lipreading	visime

ANSWERS

Matching	*Outline*	*Multiple Choice*
1. e	**1.** B	**1.** d
2. h	**2.** C	**2.** a
3. a	**3.** L	**3.** d
4. g	**4.** O	**4.** a
5. c	**5.** A	**5.** c
6. i	**6.** J	**6.** a
7. d	**7.** K	**7.** d
8. b	**8.** N	**8.** a
9. f	**9.** D	**9.** d
	10. E	**10.** b
	11. F	**11.** b
	12. G	**12.** c
	13. H	**13.** c
	14. I	**14.** a
	15. M	**15.** b
		16. d
		17. d
		18. c

THE AUDITORY NERVOUS SYSTEM

BACKGROUND

Once sound has been transformed from an acoustic signal entering the external ear canal to a mechanical-vibratory signal within the middle ear and a neuro-chemical reaction produced by the hair cells in the cochlea, it must be transmitted to and perceived by the brain before it attains meaning. The principal function of the central auditory system is found within its capacity to organize concurrent or sequential auditory input into definite patterns. The subsequent ability to comprehend and develop spoken language is primarily dependent upon the success of the entire auditory system to process speech signals.

The nerve fibers from the cochlea emerge from the modiolus to form the cochlear branch of the auditory (VIIIth cranial) nerve, which is afferent (sensory) in that it carries impulses from the cochlea to the brain. The nerve fibers arising from the cristae of the semicircular canals and the maculae of the utricle and saccule form the vestibular branch of the auditory nerve with the two branches separating at the level of the cerebellopontine angle. The vestibular system is also afferent.

The auditory nerve fibers terminate in the cochlear nuclei with the original tonotopic organization of nerve fibers continuing at this level, through the superior olivary complex, which mediates the acoustic reflex, and on into the lateral lemniscus. Impulses continue through the midbrain and thalamus, passing through the inferior colliculi and the medial geniculate bodies in the thalamus before reaching the cortex through auditory radiations. In the cortex, selective representation of frequency is still maintained, although to a lesser degree than at more peripheral levels. Once the level of the superior olivary complex is reached, both sides of the brain are involved in the transmission of auditory information—even the information that is presented by only one ear.

As stated, the auditory system is considered to be afferent, like the eyes or the skin or the nose. It is also efferent, providing inhibitory feedback by elevating the thresholds of neurons at lower stations in the auditory tract. The auditory nervous system is probably the least understood of any of the sensory systems.

Due to the intrinsic redundancies within the auditory pathways and the extrinsic redundancies within speech and language, pathologies that may interfere with the neural transmission of sound, and an individual's ability to process speech, may not show up in the results of routine audiometric measures. Most auditory tests give results that reflect primarily the first lesion reached by the stimulus (the most peripheral lesion) but can be further complicated by a more central lesion. Ruling out one anatomical area of the auditory system should not result in a diagnosis of a lesion in a specific region elsewhere.

Disorders of the auditory nervous system may include lesions of the VIIIth nerve as a result of disease, irritation, or pressure on the nerve trunk such as from acoustic tumors, lesions of the brain from head injury or cerebrovascular accidents, or auditory processing difficulties possibly secondary to mild, transitory, fluctuant hearing loss in childhood. Auditory processing deficiencies may result in lack of attention to auditory stimuli, thereby increasing distractibility, decreasing auditory discrimination and localization abilities, and making comprehension of speech more difficult. Difficulty with auditory figure-ground differentiation results in a decreased ability for selective attention.

The primary aim of behavioral measures of central function has changed over the years. While these tests were originally designed to help identify the site of lesion, this role has largely been supplanted by the more objective electrophysiological and electroacoustical measures and advances in medical imaging. Today, behavioral measures of auditory processing are more frequently employed as screening measures for potential disorders rather than as diagnostic indices. Their true value to the audiologist has evolved in their ability to describe the communication impact of auditory processing disorders. Therapeutic intervention can best be designed and implemented based upon the study of communication impact.

OBJECTIVES

1. You should know and understand the terms in the matching exercise.

2. You should be able to fill in the outline, selecting items from the list provided.

3. You should be able to label the different parts of the auditory pathways in Figure 2.1.

4. You should be able to do the matching exercise.

5. You should be able to answer the multiple-choice questions and understand the anatomy of the central auditory system as well as causes of disorders that produce sensorineural hearing loss or auditory processing difficulties.

6. You should know and understand the terms in the vocabulary list and be able to describe or define each term.

MATCHING

Match the term from the column on the right with its definition.

Definitions	*Terms*
1. ___ The base of the brain where it connects to the spinal cord	**a.** All-or-none
	b. Auditory nerve
2. ___ The gray matter on the surface of the brain	**c.** Auditory radiations
	d. Brain stem
3. ___ That part of the central auditory pathway found in the midbrain	**e.** Central nervous system
	f. Cerebellopontine angle
4. ___ The area of the brain stem that provides facilitation and inhibition of afferent stimuli	**g.** Cerebellum
	h. Cerebral cortex
5. ___ The VIIIth cranial nerve	**i.** Cochlear nucleus
6. ___ The area of the pons that connects the ventral cochlear nucleus with the lateral lemniscus	**j.** Commissure
	k. Decussation
	l. Excitation
7. ___ The bridge connecting the two hemispheres of the brain at its base	**m.** Extra-axial
	n. Glia
8. ___ Anatomical arrangement according to the best frequency of stimulation	**o.** Heschl's gyrus
	p. Inferior colliculus
	q. Inhibition
9. ___ The area of the brain receiving fibers from the ipsilateral cochlea by way of the VIIIth cranial nerve	**r.** Integration
	s. Internal auditory canal
	t. Intra-axial
10. ___ Part of the auditory pathway receiving fibers from the cochlear nucleus	**u.** Lateral lemniscus
	v. Medial geniculate body
	w. Obscure auditory dysfunction
11. ___ The theory that nerve units fire their entire electrical charge when their threshold of stimulation is reached	**x.** Olivocochlear bundle
	y. Pons
	z. Reticular formation
12. ___ The superior temporal gyrus of the brain	**aa.** Superior olivary complex
	ab. Thalamus
13. ___ Fibers in the temporal cortex received from the medial geniculate body	**ac.** Tonotopicity
	ad. Trapezoid body

14. ___ The addition of energy to stimulate a nerve unit

15. ___ The part of the brain above the pons and medulla that is responsible for equilibrium

16. ___ The crossing over of nerve fibers from one side of the brain to the other

17. ___ The passage from the inner ear to the brain stem containing the two branches of the VIIIth nerve, facial nerve, and internal auditory artery

18. ___ Arresting or restraining a neural impulse

19. ___ The portion of the auditory pathway running from the cochlear nucleus to the inferior colliculus and medial geniculate body

20. ___ A group of fibers in the brain stem that provides inhibition to the cochlear nucleus and cochlea

21. ___ The brain and spinal cord

22. ___ Connective tissue in the brain

23. ___ Within the brain stem

24. ___ The combining of different neural functions to facilitate a process

25. ___ The area in the brain base that communicates with the cortex

26. ___ The last subcortical relay station, found in the thalamus

27. ___ The junction at the base of the brain where the cerebellum, medulla, and pons communicate

28. ___ Outside of the brain stem

29. ___ Specialized nerve fibers that connect the hemispheres of the brain

30. ___ Decreased hearing abilities, primarily in adverse listening conditions, in the absence of identifiable peripheral pathology

OUTLINE

The Auditory Nerve and Central Pathways

Anatomy of the VIIIth Nerve

1. ___
2. ___
3. ___
4. ___

Waystations in the Brain Stem

5. ___
6. ___
7. ___
8. ___
9. ___

First Order Neurons

10. ___

Second Order Neurons

11. ___

Waystations in the Midbrain

12. ___
13. ___

Fibers in the Cortex

14. ___
15. ___

Disorders

16. ___
17. ___
18. ___
19. ___
20. ___
21. ___

Evaluative Measures

22. ___
23. ___
24. ___
25. ___

Select From

A. Aging
B. Auditory radiations
C. Cochlea to cochlear nucleus
D. Cochlear branch
E. Course from the cochlear nucleus
F. Dichotic digits test
G. Dorsal cochlear nucleus
H. Heschl's gyrus
I. Inferior colliculus
J. Internal auditory canal
K. Lateral lemniscus
L. Medial geniculate body
M. Multiple sclerosis
N. Myelin sheath
O. Neuritis
P. Screening test for auditory processing disorders (SCAN)
Q. Staggered spondaic word (SSW) test
R. Superior olivary complex
S. Time compressed speech
T. Trapezoid body
U. Trauma
V. Tumors
W. Ventral cochlear nucleus
X. Vestibular branch
Y. Viral infections

ACTIVITY

Label the parts of the ascending auditory pathways in Figure 2.1, selecting the terms from the list provided. Compare your labels with those at the end of this unit.

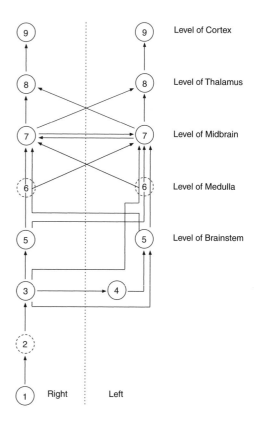

FIGURE 2.1   Ascending auditory pathways

Label

1. ___
2. ___
3. ___
4. ___
5. ___
6. ___
7. ___
8. ___
9. ___

Term

A. Auditory cortex
B. Auditory nerve (cochlear branch)
C. Cochlea
D. Cochlear nucleus (dorsal and ventral)
E. Inferior colliculus
F. Lateral lemniscus
G. Medial geniculate body
H. Superior olivary complex
I. Trapezoid body

MULTIPLE CHOICE

1. To test for central auditory disorders in a patient with normal hearing sensitivity, the audiologist will
   a. increase the extrinsic redundancy
   b. decrease the extrinsic redundancy
   c. increase the intrinsic redundancy
   d. decrease the intrinsic redundancy

2. The last subcortical relay station for auditory impulses is the
   a. inferior colliculus
   b. lateral lemniscus
   c. cochlear nucleus
   d. medial geniculate body

3. The auditory nerve is number
   a. V
   b. VI
   c. VII
   d. VIII

4. The efferent auditory system is designed for
   a. control of muscular activity
   b. feedback to lower auditory centers
   c. feedthrough to higher auditory centers
   d. work only at high intensities

5. The reticular formation is thought to aid in
   a. facilitation
   b. inhibition
   c. both a and b
   d. neither a nor b

6. The eyeblink is mediated through the
   a. superior olivary complex
   b. inferior colliculus
   c. lateral lemniscus
   d. cochlear nucleus

7. Lesions of the central auditory nervous system include
   a. tumors
   b. degenerative diseases
   c. trauma
   d. all of the above

8. Acoustic neuromas usually form
   a. on the facial nerve
   b. on the cochlear branch of the auditory nerve
   c. on the vestibular branch of the auditory nerve
   d. in the superior olivary complex

9. Crossover points uniting symmetrical portions of the two halves of the brain are called
   a. tonotopic
   b. decussations
   c. neurons
   d. none of the above

10. Fibers cross from the left cochlear nucleus to the right cochlear nucleus via the
    a. trapezoid body
    b. superior olivary complex
    c. lateral lemniscus
    d. inferior colliculus

11. The cochlear nucleus is divided into
    a. superior and inferior portions
    b. left and right portions
    c. dorsal and ventral portions
    d. none of the above

12. Impulses are transmitted from the lower brain stem to the inferior colliculus by way of the
    a. lateral lemniscus
    b. medial geniculate body
    c. thalamus
    d. auditory radiations

13. Heschl's gyrus is located in the
    a. brain stem
    b. midbrain
    c. thalamus
    d. cortex

14. Given a patient with a lesion of the left auditory nerve, a rollover on a PI/PB function would be expected in
    a. the right ear
    b. the left ear
    c. both ears
    d. neither ear

15. On auditory brain stem response (ABR) testing, a patient with a tumor of the left auditory nerve would be expected to show
    a. longer latency to wave V in the right ear than in the left ear
    b. longer latency to wave V in the left ear than in the right ear
    c. the same latency for both ears
    d. none of the above

16. Otoacoustic emissions in cases of acoustic neuroma are expected to be
    a. absent in the impaired ear, present in the normal ear
    b. present in the impaired ear, absent in the normal ear
    c. absent in the impaired ear, absent in the normal ear
    d. present in the impaired ear, present in the normal ear

17. A screening measure for retrocochlear lesion utilizing speech recognition measures repeated at a variety of sensation levels is
    a. masking-level difference
    b. Heschl's speech score
    c. performance-intensity function
    d. staggered spondaic word test

18. A disorder that creates decreased hearing abilities in noise in the absence of identifiable peripheral pathology is called
    a. auditory neuropathy
    b. obscure auditory dysfunction
    c. reticular nucleitis
    d. acoustic neuritis

19. Difficulty in language learning arising from a decrease in the size of neurons in the central auditory nervous system may be the result of
    a. masking-level differences
    b. multiple sclerosis
    c. neurofibromatosis
    d. minimal auditory deficiency syndrome

VOCABULARY

all-or-none theory	inhibition
auditory nerve	integration
auditory radiations	internal auditory canal
axon	intra-axial
brain stem	lateral lemniscus
cerebellopontine angle	medial geniculate body
central nervous system (CNS)	medulla oblongata
cerebellum	midbrain
cerebral cortex	myelin
cochlear microphonic	neuron
commissure	olivocochlear bundle
decussation	pons
dendrite	reticular formation
dorsal cochlear nucleus	second order neuron
efferent	summation
excitation	superior olivary complex
extra-axial	synapse
first order neuron	thalamus
glia	tonotopicity
Heschl's gyrus	trapezoid body
inferior colliculus	ventral cochlear nucleus

ANSWERS

Matching	*Outline*	*Activity*	*Multiple Choice*
1. d	**1.** D	**1.** C	**1.** b
2. h	**2.** J	**2.** B	**2.** d
3. p	**3.** N	**3.** D	**3.** d
4. z	**4.** X	**4.** I	**4.** b
5. b	**5.** G	**5.** H	**5.** c
6. ad	**6.** K	**6.** F	**6.** a
7. y	**7.** R	**7.** E	**7.** d
8. ac	**8.** T	**8.** G	**8.** c
9. i	**9.** W	**9.** A	**9.** b
10. aa	**10.** C		**10.** a
11. a	**11.** E		**11.** c
12. o	**12.** I		**12.** a
13. c	**13.** L		**13.** d
14. l	**14.** B		**14.** b
15. g	**15.** H		**15.** b
16. k	**16.** A		**16.** d
17. s	**17.** M		**17.** c
18. q	**18.** O		**18.** b
19. u	**19.** U		**19.** d
20. x	**20.** V		
21. e	**21.** Y		
22. n	**22.** F		
23. t	**23.** P		
24. r	**24.** Q		
25. ab	**25.** S		
26. v			
27. f			
28. m			
29. j			
30. w			

BASICS OF AUDITORY ANATOMY AND HEARING LOSS

BACKGROUND

The study of anatomy is concerned with how the body is structured, while physiology involves how it functions. To facilitate understanding, the anatomist neatly divides the mechanisms of hearing into separate compartments, at the same time realizing that these units actually function as one. The ear is made up of three portions: the outer ear, the middle ear, and the inner ear.

The outer ear is an acoustical chamber that picks up sounds from the environment and resonates at particular frequencies. At the end of the outer ear canal lies the tympanic membrane, which separates the outer ear from the middle ear. The middle ear functions in a primarily mechanical fashion, carrying vibrations to the inner ear via three tiny bones called ossicles. The inner ear is a hydromechanical system that transduces the energy it receives into neuroelectrical impulses; these impulses, in turn, transmit information about sound to the brain by way of the auditory nerve. The auditory system is usually divided in a second, different way, one that separates the combined contributions of the outer and middle ears (called the conductive mechanism) from those of the inner ear and auditory nerve (the sensorineural mechanism). Damage to the conductive mechanism causes a conductive hearing loss, and damage to the sensorineural mechanism causes a sensorineural hearing loss.

We test human hearing by two sound pathways, air conduction and bone conduction. Tests of hearing utilizing tuning forks are by no means modern, but they illustrate hearing via these two pathways (see Unit 20). Tuning-fork tests may compare the hearing of the patient to that of a presumably normal-hearing examiner, the relative sensitivity by air conduction and bone conduction, the effects on bone conduction of closing the opening into the ear, and the lateralization of sound to one ear or the other by bone conduction. The audiometer quantifies the kinds of information gleaned from tuning-fork tests so that both the type and degree of hearing loss can be determined (Unit 18).

The outer ear comprises a shell-like protrusion from each side of the head (the auricle or pinna), a tube through which sounds travel (the external auditory canal), and the eardrum membrane (more correctly called the tympanic membrane) at the end of the canal. Each middle ear consists of an air-filled space that houses the ossicles, the third of which, the stapes, is the smallest bone in the human body. The portion of the inner ear that is responsible for hearing is called the cochlea; it is filled with fluids and many microscopic components, all of which serve to convert waves into a message that travels to the base of the brain via the auditory nerve. There is a second structure in the inner ear, called the vestibule, which is responsible for balance and equilibrium. The brain stem is not coupled to the highest auditory centers in the cortex by a simple neural connection. Rather, there is a series of waystations that receive, analyze, and transmit impulses along the auditory pathway.

Any sound that courses through the outer ear, middle ear, inner ear, and beyond is heard by air conduction. It is possible to bypass the outer and middle ears by vibrating the skull mechanically and stimulating the inner ear directly. In this way the sound is heard by bone conduction. Therefore, hearing by air conduction depends on the functioning of the outer, middle, and inner ear and of the neural pathways beyond; hearing by bone conduction depends on the functioning of the inner ear and beyond.

A decrease in the strength of a sound is called attenuation. Sound attenuation is precisely the result of a conductive hearing loss. Whenever a barrier to sound is present in the outer ear or middle ear, some loss of hearing will result. Individuals will find that their sensitivity to sounds that are introduced by air conduction is impaired by such a blockage. If the sound is introduced by bone conduction, it bypasses the obstacle and goes directly to the sensorineural mechanism. Because the inner ear and the other sensorineural structures are unimpaired, the hearing by bone conduction will be normal. This impaired air conduction with normal bone conduction is the result of a conductive hearing loss. Outer ear abnormalities produce the same relationship between air and bone conduction as do abnormalities of the middle ear.

If the disturbance producing the hearing loss is situated in some portion of the sensorineural mechanism, such as the inner ear or auditory nerve, a hearing loss by air conduction will result. Because the attenuation of the sound occurs along the bone-conduction pathway, the hearing loss by bone conduction will be as great as the hearing loss by air conduction. When a hearing loss exists in which there is the same amount of attenuation for both air conduction and bone conduction, the conductive mechanism is eliminated as a possible cause of the difficulty. A diagnosis of sensorineural hearing loss can then be made. In addition to the loss of sound intensity, people with sensorineural hearing losses usually suffer from sufficient distortion as to make sounds, especially speech sounds, difficult to discriminate (Unit 19).

Problems can occur simultaneously in both the conductive and sensorineural mechanisms. This results in a loss of hearing sensitivity by bone conduction because of the sensorineural abnormality, but an even greater loss of sensitivity by air conduction due to the conductive disorder. This is true because the loss of hearing by air conduction must include the loss (by bone conduction) in the sensorineural portion plus the attenuation in the conductive portion. In other words, sound traveling on the bone-conduction pathway will be attenuated only by the defect in the inner ear or auditory nerve, but sound traveling on the air-conduction pathway will be attenuated by both conductive and sensorineural problems. This type of impairment is called a mixed hearing loss.

Some of the earliest tests of hearing probably consisted merely of producing sounds of some kind, such as clapping the hands or making vocal sounds, to see if an individual could hear them. Asking people if they could hear the ticking of a watch or the clicking of two coins together may have suggested that the examiner was attempting to sample the upper pitch range. Obviously, these tests provided little information of either a quantitative or a qualitative nature. Modern audiometry has come a long way since those days, and the diagnosis of different types of hearing loss can be accomplished today with great precision and accuracy in most cases.

OBJECTIVES

1. You should know and understand the terms in the matching exercise.

2. You should be able to fill in the outline, selecting items from the list provided.

3. You should be able to label the different parts of the auditory mechanism in Figure 3.1.

4. You should be able to answer the multiple-choice questions on the function of the ear.

5. You should know and understand the terms in the vocabulary list and be able to describe or define each term.

MATCHING

Match the term from the column on the right with its definition.

Definition   *Term*

1. ___ The sum of a combination of   **a.** Air conduction
         conductive and sensorineural
         hearing losses in the same ear   **b.** Attenuation

2. ___ Transmission of sound to the inner   **c.** Auditory
         ear by vibration of the bones of the
         skull   **d.** Auditory nerve

                                                                   e. Bone conduction
3. ___ A tone presented to both ears
         simultaneously is perceived only in   **f.** Cochlea
         the ear in which it is louder
                                                                   g. Conductive hearing Loss
4. ___ Reduction in energy
                                                                   h. Inner ear
5. ___ The course of sounds that are
         conducted to the inner ear by way   **i.** Lateralization
         of the outer and middle ear
                                                                   j. Mastoid process
6. ___ That portion of the hearing
         apparatus that converts mechanical   **k.** Middle ear
         energy to electrochemical energy
                                                                   l. Mixed hearing loss
7. ___ The bony prominence behind the
         outer ear   **m.** Outer ear

8. ___ The most external portion of the   **n.** Sensorineural hearing loss
         hearing mechanism
                                                                   o. Stenger principle
9. ___ Loss of hearing because of damage
         to the inner ear or auditory nerve

10. ___ The sense that a sound is in the right
         or left ear

11. ___ The VIIIth cranial nerve connecting
         the inner ear with the brain

12. ___ The air-filled cavity behind the
         tympanic membrane that holds the
         three smallest bones of the body

13. ___ The loss of sound sensitivity because
         of damage to the outer or middle ear

14. ___ Reference to the sense of hearing

15. ___ The portion of the inner ear
         responsible for the hearing function

OUTLINE

The Human Ear

Outer Ear

1. ___

2. ___

3. ___

Middle Ear

4. ___

5. ___

6. ___

Inner Ear

7. ___

8. ___

Auditory Nerve

9. ___

Select From

A. Air-filled space with mucous membrane lining

B. Carries impulses to the brain

C. Tympanic membrane

D. External ear canal

E. Funnel-shaped structure

F. Open air-filled space

G. Snail-like structure

H. Tiniest bones in the body

I. Transducer

ACTIVITY

Label the items in Figure 3.1. Select the terms from the list provided.

Label

1. ___

2. ___

3. ___

4. ___

5. ___

6. ___

7. ___

8. ___

Term

A. Air-conduction pathway

B. Auditory nerve

C. Bone-conduction pathway

D. Conductive mechanism

E. Inner ear

F. Middle ear

G. Outer ear

H. Sensorineural mechanism

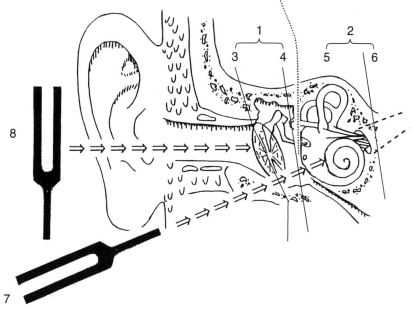

FIGURE 3.1

MULTIPLE CHOICE

1. The air-conduction pathway is the
   a. outer ear, inner ear, auditory nerve, middle ear
   b. outer ear, middle ear
   c. outer ear, middle ear, inner ear, auditory nerve
   d. inner ear, auditory nerve

2. The bone-conduction pathway is the
   a. outer ear, inner ear, auditory nerve, middle ear
   b. outer ear, middle ear
   c. outer ear, middle ear, inner ear, auditory nerve
   d. inner ear, auditory nerve

3. When air conduction is impaired and bone conduction is normal, the interpretation is
   a. conductive hearing loss
   b. mixed hearing loss
   c. normal hearing
   d. sensorineural hearing loss

4. When air conduction is impaired and bone conduction is impaired to the same degree, the interpretation is
   a. conductive hearing loss
   b. mixed hearing loss
   c. normal hearing
   d. sensorineural hearing loss

5. When air conduction is normal and bone conduction is normal, the interpretation is
   a. conductive hearing loss
   b. mixed hearing loss
   c. normal hearing
   d. sensorineural hearing loss

6. When air conduction is impaired and bone conduction is impaired, but to a lesser degree, the interpretation is
   a. conductive hearing loss
   b. mixed hearing loss
   c. normal hearing
   d. sensorineural hearing loss

7. The conductive mechanism is comprised of
   a. outer ear and middle ear
   b. middle ear and inner ear
   c. inner ear and auditory nerve
   d. auditory nerve and outer ear

8. The sensorineural mechanism is comprised of
   a. outer ear and middle ear
   b. middle ear and inner ear
   c. inner ear and auditory nerve
   d. auditory nerve and outer ear

VOCABULARY

air conduction	lateralization
attenuation	mastoid process
auditory	middle ear
auditory nerve	mixed hearing loss
bone conduction	outer ear
cochlea	sensorineural hearing loss
conductive hearing loss	Stenger principle
inner ear	

ANSWERS

Matching	*Outline*	*Activity*	*Multiple Choice*
1. l	**1.** D	**1.** D	**1.** c
2. e	**2.** E	**2.** H	**2.** d
3. o	**3.** F	**3.** G	**3.** a
4. b	**4.** A	**4.** F	**4.** d
5. a	**5.** C	**5.** E	**5.** c
6. h	**6.** H	**6.** B	**6.** b
7. j	**7.** G	**7.** C	**7.** a
8. m	**8.** I	**8.** A	**8.** c
9. n	**9.** B		
10. i			
11. d			
12. k			
13. g			
14. c			
15. f			

BONE CONDUCTION

BACKGROUND

Pure-tone bone-conduction tests are performed with an oscillator from an audiometer pressed tightly against the skull. They are carried out to determine the sensorineural sensitivity of human hearing. Their purpose is to bypass the conductive mechanisms of the outer ear and middle ear and, by distorting the skull, set the structures of the inner ear into vibration, resulting in neural transmission to the brain.

The traveling wave set up in the inner ear by bone conduction is intended to stimulate the end organ of hearing, the cochlea. Therefore, whereas air-conduction tests measure the intensity of a signal required to reach a patient's threshold of audibility, including the entire auditory system, bone-conduction tests theoretically involve only the sensorineural structures of the inner ear and the pathways beyond. These principles are often violated by certain factors, and in many cases responses to bone-conduction stimuli are modified by disorders of the outer ear and middle ear. Because both inner ears are embedded in the bones of the skull, it is virtually impossible to stimulate one without stimulating the other.

The purpose of measuring hearing by bone conduction is to determine the patient's sensorineural sensitivity. When the skull is set into vibration by a bone-conduction oscillator, the bones of the skull become distorted, resulting in distortion of the structures of hearing within the cochlea of the inner ear. This distortion activates the hair cells within the cochlea and gives rise to electrochemical activity that is identical to the activity created by an air-conduction signal. This is called distortional bone conduction.

While the skull is moving, the chain of tiny bones in the middle ear, owing to its inertia, lags behind so that the third bone, the stapes, moves in and out of the oval window that separates the middle ear from the inner ear. Thus, activity is generated within the cochlea that is identical to air-conduction stimulation. This mode of inner-ear stimulation is appropriately called inertial bone conduction.

Simultaneously, oscillation of the skull causes vibration of the column of air in the outer-ear canal. Some of these sound waves pass out of the ear, whereas others go further down the canal, vibrating the tympanic membrane, and follow the same sound route as air conduction. This third mode is called osseotympanic bone conduction. Hearing by bone conduction results from an interaction of these three modes of stimulating the cochlea.

For many years the prominent bone behind the ear (the mastoid process) has been the place on the head from which bone-conduction measurements have been made. This was probably chosen (1) because bone-conducted tones are loudest from the mastoid in normal-hearing persons and (2) because of each mastoid process's proximity to the ear being tested. Probably the bone-conducted tone is loudest from behind the ear because the chain of middle ear bones is driven on a direct axis, taking maximum advantage of its hinged action. The notion that placing an oscillator behind the right ear results in stimulation of only the right cochlea is false because vibration of the skull from any location results in approximately equal stimulation of both cochleas.

It has been demonstrated that the forehead is in many ways superior to the mastoid process for measurement of clinical bone-conduction thresholds. Variations produced by oscillator-to-skull pressure, artifacts created by abnormalities of the sound-conducting mechanism of the middle ear, test-retest differences, and so on are all of smaller consequence when testing from the forehead than from the mastoid. It has been shown that the greater amount of acoustic energy generated in the outer ear canal when the mastoid is the test site, as compared to the forehead, is further evidence of the advantage of forehead testing.

In addition to the theoretical advantages of forehead bone-conduction, there are numbers of practical conveniences. The headband used to hold the bone-conduction oscillator is much easier to affix to the head than the mastoid headband. Also, eyeglasses need not be removed when the oscillator is placed on the forehead, which is the case for mastoid placement.

The main disadvantage of testing from the forehead is that about 10 dB greater intensity is required to stimulate normal thresholds, resulting in a decrease of the maximum level at which testing can be carried out. Although bone-conduction testing should sometimes be done from both the forehead and the mastoid, the forehead is preferable for routine audiometry. Despite negative reports on mastoid test accuracy and other problems that go back many years, the mastoid process continues to be the preferred bone-conduction oscillator site among audiologists.

When the mastoid is the place of measurement, a steel headband crosses the top of the head. If testing is to be done from the forehead, the bone-conduction oscillator should be affixed to the centerline of the skull, just above the eyebrow line. A strap encircles the head, holding the oscillator in place. All interfering hair must be pushed out of the way, and the concave side of the oscillator should be placed against the skull.

Bone-conduction tests often present insurmountable difficulties in some patients, although a competent audiologist can find clever ways around many of these difficulties. Despite their problems, there is no evidence that bone-conduction audiometry will be replaced by other measures of sensorineural sensitivity. However, when the absence of any conductive hearing loss can be clearly documented, such as when tympanograms are normal and acoustic reflexes are present, many clinicians believe that bone-conduction testing can be foregone in routine audiometrics.

OBJECTIVES

1. You should know and understand the terms in the matching exercise.

2. You should be able to fill in the outline, selecting items from the list provided.

3. You should understand the principles of bone-conduction tests, why these tests are performed, and why they may not always achieve their objectives.

4. You should be able to answer the multiple-choice questions and grasp the fundamental concepts of bone conduction.

5. You should know and understand the terms in the vocabulary list and be able to describe or define each term.

MATCHING

Match the term from the column on the right with its definition.

Definition

1. ___ The mode of bone conduction involving the middle ear

2. ___ A test of lateralization performed by placing the bone-conduction vibrator on the forehead

3. ___ Introduction of noise into the nontest ear to eliminate cross-hearing

4. ___ The mode of bone conduction involving the outer ear

5. ___ The mode of bone conduction involving only the inner ear

6. ___ The increase in the loudness of bone-conducted tones that occurs when the ear is occluded

7. ___ A device used for calibrating the bone-conduction system of an audiometer

8. ___ Responses to bone-conducted stimuli that have been felt by the patient rather than heard

Term

a. Artificial mastoid

b. Audiometric Weber

c. Distortional

d. Inertial

e. Masking

f. Occlusion effect

g. Osseotympanic

h. Tactile

OUTLINE

Bone Conduction

Outer-Ear Effects

   1. ___

   2. ___

Middle-Ear Effects

   3. ___

   4. ___

Inner-Ear Effects

   5. ___

   6. ___

   7. ___

   8. ___

Vibrator Placement
Mastoid Advantage

   9. ___

Mastoid Disadvantages

   10. ___

   11. ___

   12. ___

Forehead Advantages

   13. ___

   14. ___

Forehead Disadvantage

   15. ___

Air-Bone Relationships

   16. ___

   17. ___

Occlusion Effect

   18. ___

Cross Hearing

   19. ___

   20. ___

Select From

A. Affected more by middle-ear conditions

B. Air pressure in middle ear

C. Distortion of temporal bone

D. Effects of covering the ear

E. Energy in outer ear canal

F. Poorer (higher) auditory threshold

G. Improved test reliability

H. Interaural attenuation

I. Intertest variability

J. Less affected by vibrator pressure

K. Better (lower) auditory threshold

L. Masking

M. More affected by vibrator pressure

N. Ossicular chain impedance

O. Oval window release

P. Poorer test reliability

Q. Round window release

R. Shearing of hair cells

S. Tactile response

T. Tympanic membrane impedance

MULTIPLE CHOICE

1. During bone-conduction testing, low-frequency sounds appear louder when the ear is covered because of
   a. masking
   b. the occlusion effect
   c. the Rinne effect
   d. cross-hearing

2. The mode of bone conduction affected by the outer ear is
   a. osseotympanic
   b. inertial
   c. distortional
   d. compressional

3. Interaural attenuation for bone conduction is generally considered to be ___ dB
   a. 0
   b. 25
   c. 50
   d. 75

4. Intertest variability may cause
   a. AC = BC
   b. AC > BC
   c. AC < BC
   d. all of the above

5. The occlusion effect is found at ___ Hz
   a. 250
   b. 250, 500
   c. 250, 500, 1000
   d. 250, 500, 1000, 2000

6. Testing bone conduction from the forehead requires ___ voltage to produce a response than testing from the mastoid
   a. more
   b. less
   c. the same

7. Forehead placement of the bone-conduction vibrator reduces the ___ mode of bone conduction
   a. inertial
   b. osseotympanic
   c. distortional
   d. compressional

8. The column of air in the external auditory meatus plays a large role in the ___ mode of bone conduction
   a. distortional
   b. osseotympanic
   c. inertial
   d. compressional

9. Advantages of testing bone conduction from the forehead over the mastoid include
   a. less effect of middle-ear disorders
   b. higher intensity required for threshold
   c. lower tactile thresholds
   d. greater interaural attenuation

10. To increase interaural attenuation when masking for bone conduction, one may use
   a. insert receivers
   b. supra-aural receivers
   c. sound field
   d. a hearing aid

11. False air-bone gaps may not be produced by
   a. collapsing ear canals
   b. tactile bone-conduction responses
   c. contralateral bone-conduction responses
   d. distortional bone conduction

12. A profound bilateral sensorineural hearing loss might look like a mixed loss because
   a. cross-hearing is taking place
   b. bone-conduction responses are tactile
   c. ambient noise levels are too high
   d. improper masking is used

13. The mode of bone conduction affected by the inner ear is
    a. fractional
    b. unknown
    c. distortional
    d. osseotympanic

14. The impedance of the ossicular chain plays an important role in the ___ mode of bone conduction
    a. osseotympanic
    b. distortional
    c. inertial
    d. compressional

15. As frequency increases, the occlusion effect
    a. decreases
    b. increases
    c. remains unchanged
    d. decreases, then increases

16. In testing by bone conduction with the vibrator on the right mastoid process, the sound may be heard in
    a. the right ear
    b. the left ear
    c. both ears
    d. all of the above

VOCABULARY

air-bone gap
artificial mastoid
Carhart notch
compressional bone conduction
cross hearing
distortional bone conduction

inertial bone conduction
insert receiver
interaural attenuation
masking
occlusion effect
osseotympanic bone conduction

ANSWERS

Matching	*Outline*	*Multiple Choice*
1. d	**1.** E	**1.** b
2. b	**2.** T	**2.** a
3. e	**3.** B	**3.** a
4. g	**4.** N	**4.** d
5. c	**5.** C	**5.** c
6. f	**6.** O	**6.** a
7. a	**7.** Q	**7.** a
8. h	**8.** R	**8.** b
	9. K	**9.** a
	10. A	**10.** a
	11. M	**11.** d
	12. P	**12.** b
	13. G	**13.** c
	14. J	**14.** c
	15. F	**15.** a
	16. I	**16.** d
	17. S	
	18. D	
	19. H	
	20. L	

EDUCATING CHILDREN WITH HEARING LOSS

BACKGROUND

A variety of legislation has been enacted for improved education of children with disabilities following the establishment of the Bureau of Education of the Handicapped in 1966. To meet the spirit of the law for each of these important legislations, audiologists must not only identify, assess, and plan intervention for children with hearing loss, but they must also be familiar with general education curriculum standards, goals, and benchmarks, as well as the support systems that children with hearing loss may need to attain their highest levels of achievement.

Early intervention services include audiology, speech-language pathology, case management, family training, health services, nutrition, occupational therapy, physical therapy, psychological and social services, transportation, and more. In all states, children who are suspected of having a hearing loss are entitled to free testing. The purpose, of course, is to identify, as early as possible, those children who require special assistance.

Following passage of the Education for All Handicapped Children Act (PL 94-142) many children have been mainstreamed, resulting in education within the regular classroom except for times specifically designed for them to receive support services related to their disabilities. As a result, large numbers of children with profound hearing losses were moved away from specialized schools for the deaf, and many of these schools began to close as a consequence. It is unfortunate that the requirement of education within the "least restrictive environment" was interpreted as endorsing mainstreaming for *all* children. Restrictive environments may be more appropriately defined as settings that limit a child's classroom potential, and the least restrictive environment as that environment most appropriate for the individual child.

Childhood hearing loss delays the development of receptive and expressive communication skills, creating learning problems that reduce academic performance, produce social isolation, lower self-concept, and restrict future vocational options. Children who are born with or acquire a hearing loss before they develop speech and language are said to be prelinguistically hearing impaired. The proper methods of educating children with a severe hearing handicap are not agreed upon, even among the most well-meaning experts. One group believes that the "Deaf" should be considered as a group unto themselves with no attempt made to integrate them educationally into a hearing environment. These people are often committed to one of several forms of manual communication. A second group believes that children should be taught speech at all costs, taking maximum advantage of residual hearing through amplification, and should use no signs whatever. Still others believe in a combined approach of simultaneously speaking and signing known as total communication. Regardless of the preferred method, there is universal agreement that the earlier the hearing loss is detected, and steps taken toward educating the child, the better the prognosis for the development of language at an early age and the achievement of the highest possible educational attainment.

A variety of placement options may be available for the formal education of children with hearing loss. These include privately and publicly funded institutions, residential and day schools, and public schools. Given the emphasis on mainstream education, children with hearing loss comprise the largest group requiring special educational considerations in the regular classroom. Even so, classroom teachers often admit to an inadequate knowledge base for the proper education and management of students with hearing loss. In addition to educational management, teachers must have information about classroom acoustics, individually worn amplification devices, and systems to help improve the signal-to-noise ratios for children.

Educational placement decisions for the child with hearing loss may be one of the most stressing and difficult management situations parents must face. The placement a parent decides upon may change over time based on the child's performance in the setting selected and new information acquired. Audiologists must be prepared to facilitate families skillfully as they implement these important decisions so critical to the development of the child with hearing loss.

OBJECTIVES

1. You should know and understand the terms in the matching exercise.

2. You should be able to fill in the outline, selecting items from the list provided.

3. You should understand the methods, advantages, and disadvantages of the manual approaches to educating children with hearing impairments.

4. You should understand the methods, advantages, and disadvantages of the oral approaches to educating children with hearing impairments.

5. You should understand the methods, advantages, and disadvantages of the combined approaches to educating children with hearing impairments.

6. You should be able to answer the multiple-choice questions on pediatric management.

7. You should know and understand the terms in the vocabulary list and be able to describe or define each term.

MATCHING

Match the term from the column on the right with its definition.

Definition

1. ___ The use of hand signs and facial and body movements in communicating with persons with a hearing impairment

2. ___ A method of manual communication that follows English word order but is relatively uncommon

3. ___ Writing in the air with the fingers to spell out words

4. ___ Using hand signs with specific signs for articles and verbs

5. ___ A unisensory approach to teaching children with severe hearing loss that relies solely on hearing

6. ___ A less than normally rigid system of signs

7. ___ Educating individuals with hearing impairment to maximize auditory cues, often utilizing drilling exercises

8. ___ Educating children in the least restrictive environment

9. ___ A multisensory approach to teaching speech

Term

a. American Sign Language

b. Auditory training

c. Auditory-verbal training

d. Aural/Oral

e. Fingerspelling

f. Linguistics of Visual English

g. Mainstreaming

h. Signing Essential English

i. Signing Exact English

OUTLINE

Educating Children with Hearing Loss

Goals

1. ___

2. ___

3. ___

4. ___

5. ___

Assessment

6. ___

7. ___

8. ___

9. ___

Communication Skills

10. ___

11. ___

12. ___

13. ___

Communication Systems

14. ___

15. ___

16. ___

17. ___

18. ___

19. ___

20. ___

21. ___

22. ___

Select From

A. American Sign Language

B. Auditory Global Method

C. Auditory training

D. Educational achievement

E. Educational potential

F. Fingerspelling

G. Integration into Deaf society

H. Integration into hearing society

I. Intelligence

J. Language

K. Language concepts

L. Linguistics of Visual English

M. Multisensory stimulation

N. Personality

O. Psychological potential

P. Seeing Essential English

Q. Signing Exact English

R. Social potential

S. Speech

T. Speechreading

U. Systematic sign language

V. Total Communication

MULTIPLE CHOICE

1. The sign system about which most information is known is
    a. ASL
    b. LOVE
    c. SEE1
    d. AMESLISH

2. All elements of English grammar may be included in
    a. LOVE
    b. SEE1
    c. fingerspelling
    d. ASL

3. The least extensive sign system in terms of vocabulary is
    a. ASL
    b. LOVE
    c. SEE1
    d. SEE2

4. Signing and speaking simultaneously is called
    a. ASL
    b. total communication
    c. visual communication
    d. SEE3

5. A generic term describing hearing disability regardless of degree is
    a. hearing impaired
    b. hard of hearing
    c. deaf
    d. deafened

6. Children with hearing losses in the 70 to 90 dB HL range, without amplification, may be expected to
    a. have difficulty mainly with faint speech
    b. understand conversation at distances less than 5 feet
    c. understand speech only if speakers raise their voices
    d. identify loud sounds near the ear and perhaps a few vowel sounds

7. Given appropriate training and amplification, success may usually be achieved in regular schools by children with hearing losses up to
    a. 30 dB HL
    b. 50 dB HL

    c. 70 dB HL

    d. 90 dB HL

8. Without universal newborn hearing screening, early identification is most likely for a child with a hearing loss of

    a. 20 dB HL

    b. 40 dB HL

    c. 60 dB HL

    d. 80 dB HL

9. The auditory-verbal method of training children who have hearing impairments

    a. insists on auditory cues exclusively

    b. insists on visual cues exclusively

    c. combines visual with auditory cues

    d. none of the above

10. Public Law 94-142 mandates that

    a. all handicapped children must be educated in regular classrooms

    b. all children who have hearing impairments must be educated in regular classrooms

    c. all children must be educated in the least restrictive environment

    d. children with hearing losses greater than 90 dB HL must be educated in special classrooms

11. The auditory verbal method states that

    a. the exclusive teaching channel should be auditory

    b. the primary teaching channel should be auditory

    c. the primary teaching channel should be visual

    d. the same teaching methods should be used all over the world

12. Many experts feel that integration of a child with hearing impairment into a regular classroom is best achieved with a teaching method involving

    a. fingerspelling

    b. signing

    c. auditory-oral

    d. none of the above

13. The intelligence of young children who have severe hearing impairments is best determined by tests that

    a. rely heavily on language

    b. rely lightly on language

    c. rely heavily on performance

    d. include fingerspelling for instruction

14. Assessing personality in young children who cannot hear is difficult because
    a. tests are complicated by vocabulary items
    b. personality development is related closely to language development
    c. emotional immaturity is caused by frustration in some children
    d. all of the above

15. Teaching children who cannot hear to speak involves senses that are
    a. tactile
    b. kinesthetic
    c. visual
    d. all of the above

16. Children who are prelinguistically hearing impaired are not those who
    a. lose hearing shortly after birth
    b. are born with hearing loss
    c. lose hearing before they learn language
    d. lose hearing after they learn language

17. Teaching systems for children who cannot hear that include vision, hearing, tactile, and kinesthetic senses are called
    a. unisensory
    b. auditory verbal
    c. multisensory
    d. ASL

18. Auditory training may take advantage of
    a. wearable hearing aids
    b. magnetic loop systems
    c. FM carrier systems
    d. all of the above

19. Speechreading is usually taught to children
    a. in isolation
    b. in combination with other lessons
    c. without amplification
    d. in darkened areas to increase concentration

20. Many experts agree that children with hearing losses sufficient to require hearing aids should be fitted
    a. when the child can care for the instrument
    b. at the age when children normally begin to speak
    c. at the earliest possible time regardless of age
    d. when the child reaches school age

VOCABULARY

acoupedic method	mainstreaming
American Sign Language (ASL)	multisensory stimulation
auditory-aural	Signing Essential English (SEE$_1$)
auditory global method	Signing Exact English (SEE$_2$)
auditory training	speechreading
aural-oral	systematic sign language
fingerspelling	total communication (TC)
Linguistics of Visual English (LOVE)	unisensory stimulation

ANSWERS

Matching	*Outline*	*Multiple Choice*
1. a	1. E	1. a
2. f	2. G	2. c
3. e	3. H	3. b
4. h	4. O	4. b
5. c	5. R	5. a
6. i	6. D	6. d
7. b	7. I	7. d
8. g	8. K	8. d
9. d	9. N	9. a
	10. C	10. c
	11. J	11. a
	12. S	12. c
	13. T	13. c
	14. A	14. d
	15. B	15. d
	16. F	16. d
	17. L	17. c
	18. M	18. d
	19. P	19. b
	20. Q	20. c
	21. U	
	22. V	

▪ ▪ ▪ ▪ ▪

HEARING INSTRUMENTS AND ASSISTIVE LISTENING DEVICES

BACKGROUND

Amplification and sensory systems—either personal, in the form of hearing aids or implants, or supplemental, in the form of assistive devices such as television amplifiers—comprise a major component of management endeavors for the patient with hearing loss. Although it is true that some patients cannot use or do not desire hearing aids, amplification should be considered for all patients with hearing impairment as part of a total rehabilitation program. It was not until the late nineteenth century that the first electric hearing aid was produced. Nearly forty years later the development of the vacuum tube and then the transistor allowed for significant miniaturization and the advent of head-worn amplification with an increased frequency bandwidth. Today's hearing aids can be small enough to be well hidden deep in the external ear canal with digital signal processing that alters amplification characteristics with lightning-fast speed as listening demands change. In addition to the advantages of digital processing, directional microphones are becoming increasingly popular for improving signal-to-noise ratio. Many hearing aids also contain electromagnetic coils (known as t-coils or audiocoils) for enhanced use of the telephone and access to a variety of assistive listening devices.

Acoustic characteristics of hearing aids are usually described in terms of their output sound-pressure level (OSPL; the maximum power output that can be delivered regardless of the strength of the input signal), acoustic gain (the difference in decibels between the input and output sound-pressure levels), and the frequency response (range and output of frequencies amplified). The American National Standards Institute (ANSI) sets specifications for hearing aids' electroacoustic properties, which are measured in a coupler the size of an average adult ear canal (2 cubic centimeters) attached to a microphone. Hearing aids are selected for patients with hearing loss based upon the electroacoustic properties of the instruments, the style appropriate for the degree of hearing loss and the abilities of the individual to handle various sizes of hearing aids, and the listening demands the individual confronts in daily life.

A variety of prescription methods are currently employed by audiologists to match, as closely as possible, the acoustic characteristics of the earmold and hearing aid to the acoustic needs of the patient. In addition to more sophisticated electroacoustic circuit modifications than previously available, through venting and special earmold designs, low-frequency energy can be deemphasized for patients with hearing losses that are primarily in the higher frequencies. Mid-frequency energy can be modified with acoustic dampers or filters in the tubing of the earmolds or ear hooks of the aids, and high-frequency energy can be enhanced with bell-shaped tubing or belled receiver openings.

When air conduction hearing aids are not a viable option due to pinna or external ear canal abnormalities or active ear infection, bone-conduction hearing aids may be the instruments of choice. A number of implantable hearing aids are available for audiological management, including cochlear implants that directly stimulate the auditory nerve when no other form of acoustic amplification provides benefit. The degree of success with cochlear implantation hinges on a variety of personal and support factors, but generally adults with postlinguistic deafness of shorter duration and children implanted before 2 years of age attain the highest levels of success.

Regardless of the type of amplification selected for a patient, measures should be made to verify that the results obtained closely approximate the expected outcome and that the benefit received is recognized as a valid improvement by the user. Verification of hearing aid performance is frequently obtained through probe-microphone measures using a small silicone tube that is attached to a microphone and placed in the patient's ear canal. Such measures for validation are much more accurate than the electroacoustic measures taken in a 2 cc coupler, which is required for verification that an instrument meets manufacturer specifications, as the former account for the personal ear canal resonance characteristics of the individual. Validation of hearing aid fittings is frequently obtained through the use of self-assessment questionnaires often given pre- and post-hearing aid fitting.

Following the hearing aid fitting it is the audiologist's responsibility to ensure that patients, and often family members or parents, are familiar with the needed care and maintenance of these electronic devices. Some patients need additional counseling from the audiologist prior to the hearing aid selection process to help them accept the impact of the hearing loss and their own responsibilities toward improving the communication difficulties they face.

One of the major disadvantages of wearable hearing aids is the environmental noise that exists between the microphones of the hearing aids and the talker, which creates adverse signal-to-noise ratios and decreased speech intelligibility. In addition, the restoration of hearing loss obtained through amplification is typically limited to only one-half of the hearing loss itself, primarily due to tolerance problems inherent in many hearing losses. To further remediate the effects of hearing loss, a variety of assistive listening devices and vibratory or visual alerting technologies may be employed.

OBJECTIVES

1. You should know and understand the terms in the matching exercise.

2. You should be able to fill in the outline, selecting items from the list provided.

3. You should know and be able to identify the components of a hearing aid.

4. You should understand the implications of assistive listening devices.

5. You should be able to answer the multiple-choice questions about hearing instruments.

6. You should know and understand the terms in the vocabulary list and be able to describe or define each term.

MATCHING

Match the term from the column on the right with its definition.

Definition

1. ___ A device surgically placed in the inner ear for persons with profound hearing loss

2. ___ The squeal that occurs when sound that is amplified and fed through the speaker of a hearing aid is picked up again by the microphone and reamplified

3. ___ An amplification system that stores and processes the input signal as sets of binary digits that represent frequency, intensity, and temporal patterns of the signal

4. ___ A device that amplifies sound and delivers it to the surface of the skin so that the different patterns of vibration can be felt

5. ___ Measurements made of sound-pressure level in the external ear canal that show the performance characteristics of a hearing aid

6. ___ Signaling or alerting devices, in addition to hearing aids, that assist individuals with a hearing loss

7. ___ An electromagnetic device in a hearing aid that allows the user to bypass the microphone when talking on the telephone

8. ___ Hearing aids worn in both ears

9. ___ The highest sound pressure that can emit from a hearing aid regardless of the input intensity

10. ___ The custom-made device, usually made of plastic, that couples a behind-the-ear or body hearing aid to the ear

11. ___ A system for limiting the sound intensity emitted by a hearing aid by using electronic feedback circuits

12. ___ Connection to the space between the medial end of an earmold or hearing aid casing and the tympanic membrane so that a sound in that space can be measured

13. ___ The range from the lowest to the highest frequency amplified by a hearing aid

14. ___ A specified average increase of the intensity of a sound produced by a hearing aid as measured in a hearing aid test box

15. ___ The difference, in decibels, between the input intensity and the output intensity of a hearing aid

16. ___ Distortion in a hearing aid produced by the generation of overtones

17. ___ Another term for automatic gain control

18. ___ Hearing aid gain obtained through probe-microphone measures

Term

a. Acoustic feedback

b. Acoustic gain

c. Automatic gain control

d. Binaural hearing aids

e. Cochlear implant

f. Compression amplification

g. Digital hearing aid

h. Earmold

i. Frequency response

j. Harmonic distortion

k. Hearing assistance technologies/Assistive listening devices

l. Output sound pressure level (OSPL)

m. Probe tube

n. Real ear insertion gain (REIG)

o. Real ear measurements

p. Reference test gain

q. Telecoil

r. Vibrotactile hearing aid

OUTLINE

Hearing Aids

Types

1. ___
2. ___
3. ___
4. ___
5. ___
6. ___
7. ___
8. ___
9. ___

Characteristics

10. ___
11. ___
12. ___
13. ___
14. ___
15. ___

Components

16. ___
17. ___
18. ___
19. ___
20. ___
21. ___
22. ___
23. ___
24. ___

Select From

A. Air conduction
B. Amplifier
C. Battery
D. Behind-the-ear
E. Body worn
F. Bone conduction
G. Completely in-the-canal
H. Cord
I. CROS
J. Digital processor
K. Earmold
L. Eyeglass
M. Frequency response
N. Gain
O. Harmonic distortion
P. Intermodulation distortion
Q. In-the-canal
R. In-the-ear
S. Microphone
T. OSPL
U. Peak clipping
V. Telephone pickup (telecoil)
W. Tone control
X. Volume control

MULTIPLE CHOICE

1. The maximum sound-pressure level emitted from the receiver of a hearing aid, regardless of its input level is called
   a. acoustic gain
   b. OSPL
   c. frequency response
   d. distortion

2. The difference, in decibels, between the input level of a sound source and the amplified response of a hearing aid is its
   a. acoustic gain
   b. OSPL
   c. frequency response
   d. distortion

3. A sweep frequency audio oscillator is used to determine a hearing aid's
   a. distortion
   b. OSPL
   c. frequency response
   d. b and c

4. Lack of sound coming from a hearing aid may be caused by
   a. occluded ear mold
   b. twisted tubing
   c. a broken receiver
   d. all of the above

5. Acoustic feedback will not be caused by
   a. a loosely fitting earmold
   b. a twisted cord
   c. a loose connection between earmold and receiver
   d. an improperly inserted earmold

6. Weak but audible sound coming from a hearing aid will not be caused by a
   a. partially obstructed earmold
   b. weak battery
   c. switch set to "telephone" setting
   d. partially obstructed tubing

7. The input transducer of a hearing aid is its
   a. battery
   b. microphone
   c. loudspeaker
   d. volume control

8. "Ceramic," "magnetic," "dynamic," and "electret" are different kinds of
   a. loudspeakers
   b. hearing aids
   c. microphones
   d. volume controls

9. Deemphasis of different portions of the frequency response of a hearing aid may be accomplished by
   a. earmold modification
   b. internal tone adjustments
   c. changing receivers
   d. all of the above

10. Bone-conduction hearing aids are usually reserved for patients who have
    a. sensorineural hearing loss
    b. conductive hearing losses caused by otosclerosis
    c. conductive hearing losses with chronic ear drainage
    d. mixed hearing losses without chronic ear drainage

11. Acoustic feedback problems with hearing aids will not be lessened by
    a. cupping a hand behind the aided ear
    b. increasing the distance from microphone to receiver
    c. fabricating a tighter earmold
    d. replacing a cracked or damaged earmold tubing

12. Binaural amplification will often
    a. improve hearing in noise
    b. improve localization abilities
    c. decrease the effects of sensory deprivation
    d. all of the above

13. Persons with total unilateral hearing losses are sometimes helped by a hearing aid called
    a. CROS
    b. IROS
    c. NITTS
    d. ROSS

14. Cochlear implants are
    a. totally placed within the middle ear
    b. limited to use with children who have prelinguistic hearing loss
    c. effective for some recipients for telephone conversations
    d. none of the above

VOCABULARY

acoustic feedback

acoustic gain

acoustic output

automatic gain control (AGC)

binaural hearing aids

compression amplification

contralateral routing of off-side
    signals (CROS)

earmold

frequency response

harmonic distortion

hearing aid

hearing aid evaluation

Hearing Aid Industry Conference
    (HAIC)

intermodulation distortion

ringing

saturation sound pressure level
    (SSPL)

ANSWERS

Matching	*Outline*	*Multiple Choice*
1. e	**1.** A	**1.** b
2. a	**2.** D	**2.** a
3. g	**3.** E	**3.** c
4. r	**4.** F	**4.** d
5. o	**5.** G	**5.** b
6. k	**6.** I	**6.** c
7. q	**7.** L	**7.** b
8. d	**8.** Q	**8.** c
9. l	**9.** R	**9.** d
10. h	**10.** M	**10.** c
11. c	**11.** N	**11.** a
12. m	**12.** O	**12.** d
13. i	**13.** P	**13.** a
14. p	**14.** T	**14.** d
15. b	**15.** U	
16. j	**16.** B	
17. f	**17.** C	
18. n	**18.** H	
	19. J	
	20. K	
	21. S	
	22. V	
	23. W	
	24. X	

HEARING TESTS FOR CHILDREN

BACKGROUND

There is no argument about whether hearing loss in children should be detected as early and accurately as possible. What is in debate are the means, methods, accuracy, and cost-effectiveness of different approaches. Although by age 4 or 5 years, many young children can take adult hearing tests that have been only slightly modified, others require special procedures and special equipment. No hearing test on a noncooperative child is foolproof, so a battery of procedures is best advised when diagnosis is critical. Since the prevalence of hearing loss is growing, the need for pediatric audiology is self-evident.

While pediatric audiology can be stimulating and rewarding, it can also be time-consuming and frustrating. Often clinicians do not have the feeling, as they have with most adults, of complete closure on a case at the end of a diagnostic session. Nevertheless, the proper identification and management of hearing loss in children is one of the most solemn responsibilities of the audiologist. Truly, work with children is often carried out more as an art than a science, testing the cleverness and perseverance of clinicians and calling on all their training and experience. Hearing testing is designed to determine the nature and extent of a child's communicative problem and is virtually useless unless some (re)habilitative path is pursued (Unit 1). Pediatric audiology includes the use of those tests and diagnostic procedures designed especially for children who cannot be tested by conventional audiometry. Approaches vary with both the chronological and mental ages of children. Some tests, designed merely to elicit some sort of startle reaction, may be carried out on children as young as several hours of age.

Procedures that seek a startle response from a child include presenting a loud sound and observing the Moro reflex, an overall embracing reaction. The auropalpebral reflex (APR) is a contraction of the ring of muscles around the eyes that appears like an eye blink when a loud sound is heard. Some clinicians find a procedure called behavioral observation audiometry (BOA) useful by looking for any kind of increase, decrease, or cessation of ongoing activity seen in a baby or young child.

Some procedures require that a child look in the direction of a sound source. In children with normal hearing or equal amounts of hearing loss in both ears sound localization is normally in place by age 6 months. One such test that has enjoyed popularity for more than four decades is the conditioned orientation reflex (COR). With this test, a child is placed facing and between two loudspeakers. The child, often seated on a caregiver's or assistant's lap, is in the right angle corner of a right triangle with two loudspeakers placed at the other two (45 degree) angles. The child's attention is directed forward, between the two loudspeakers and when a loud sound, such as a warble tone, is emitted from one speaker, a visual stimulus (e.g., flashing light, animated toy, computer graphic, etc.) also appears briefly from that site, which causes the child to look in the direction of the sound source. A number of pairings of sound and flashing light often results in the child's looking to the source of the sound in search of the visual reinforcement. Once this conditioning has taken place, the intensity of the signal is lowered and threshold is sought. While it is reasonable to expect adults and older children to give responses close to their auditory thresholds, it is unwise to assume that the lowest level at which a child responds is his or her actual threshold. There are many obvious explanations for this. The term minimum response level (MRL) has been coined to describe the responses given by children; how close this is to their actual thresholds is often unknown until several tests have been completed.

Play audiometry is a tried-and-true procedure. Many children will play a game wherein they observe adults (and caregivers and older siblings, if those can be included) who sit around, often on the floor of the sound suite, holding something like a soft plastic block next to one ear. Every time a loud tone is introduced, everyone throws his or her block into a bucket, and a lot of smiling and clapping follows. Most children will get excited at this game and grab another block and throw it. The block should be returned to the child and the listening postures resumed. The child receives the social reward when he or she follows suit and throws a block only when a tone is on. Once the patient learns the task, the child is allowed to go first with the response.

Anything that results in the child's giving a response is acceptable. While some young children will accept earphones, many will not, and the testing may be done in the sound field, introducing tones through one or more loudspeakers. When sound-field audiometry is done, there is no way to know which ear is hearing the stimuli. However, often after the task is learned and enjoyed by the child, transition to earphones is not difficult.

Some of the principles of classical conditioning have been applied to the testing of children's hearing. Basically, conditioning consists of a stimulus, a response, and a reinforcer to encourage repetition of the response. In pediatric audiometry the stimulus is often a pure tone, a response may be a child encouraged to press a button, and the reinforcer something that will please or amuse the child. It is known that tangible reinforcers, like food or a token the child is allowed to keep, usually work better than intangible reinforcers like praise or the clapping of hands. Reinforcement works best when it is delivered immediately after the response, which is why mechanical devices dedicated to this purpose often work so well. A number of techniques and devices have been developed, including one called tangible reinforcement operant conditioning audiometry (TROCA), wherein a candy pellet is delivered via a chute each time a child correctly indicates that a tone has been heard.

If a child has any verbal vocabulary, even if it is only receptive, it is helpful to try to obtain an SRT. This can be done by having a child point to or pick up a picture or object. Ideally, spondaic words should be used but it has been shown that children's thresholds with monosyllabic words are quite similar to SRTs obtained with spondees. Speech-recognition scores may be obtained with modified versions of adult tests, like the use of PB word lists or with picture-pointing tests for children who have enough vocabulary but whose verbal responses are unacceptable for some reason.

Most audiologists would agree that the testing of children's hearing presents a number of difficult and unique challenges. It is usual for two clinicians to participate in these pediatric examinations, or the assistance of a parent may be sought. Often it is necessary to accept small amounts of information about a child's hearing, so it is quite common for a diagnosis to require a number of attempts.

Still other procedures involve objective tests that measure changes in electrophysiological states or electroacoustical properties in response to sound, or the detection of sounds emitted from the ear (Unit 14). With the advent of universal newborn hearing screening, the first hearing test a child receives is often one of these objective measures. While these and many of the behavioral measures used in pediatric audiology provide insights into hearing problems that children might have, the pure-tone audiogram remains the gold standard. Until that has been obtained, hearing testing is incomplete. When children are old enough to take pure-tone tests, that is a good place to begin.

OBJECTIVES

1. You should know and understand the terms in the matching exercise.

2. You should be able to fill in the outline, selecting items from the list provided.

3. You should know which hearing tests to use with children of different ages or different levels of function.

4. You should know what special equipment is necessary for specific tests.

5. You should be able to answer the multiple-choice questions on pediatric diagnosis.

6. You should know and understand the terms in the vocabulary list and be able to describe or define each term.

MATCHING

Match the term from the column on the right with its definition.

Definition

1. ___ A set of criteria designed to help identify infants and young children at risk for hearing loss

2. ___ A system for checking the reliability of screening measures

3. ___ Observation of changes in the behavior of small children in response to sound

4. ___ A nonlinguistic speech audiometric measurement for assessing audibility of the acoustics of speech

5. ___ The use of tangible reinforcement to condition young children to take a hearing test

6. ___ The use of a light or picture to reinforce a child's response to sound.

7. ___ The use of games or other play techniques in teaching children to respond during hearing tests

8. ___ A sound-field hearing test for children involving localization of the sound with visual reinforcement for head turning

9. ___ A form of conditioned audiometry using tangible reinforcers, such as food or tokens

10. ___ A startle response to sound in the form of an embracing movement

11. ___ Contraction of the muscles around the eyes in response to a loud sound

12. ___ The child's lowest level response (not necessarily the threshold) to an acoustic stimulus

Term

a. Auropalpebral reflex

b. Behavioral observation audiometry

c. Conditioned orientation reflex

d. High-risk registry

e. Ling six-sound test

f. Minimum response level

g. Moro reflex

h. Operant conditioning audiometry

i. Play audiometry

j. Tetrachoric table

k. TROCA

l. Visual reinforcement audiometry

OUTLINE

Pediatric Diagnosis

Testing Infants

 1. ___

 2. ___

 3. ___

Testing Infants and Small Children

 4. ___

 5. ___

 6. ___

 7. ___

 8. ___

Testing Older Children (Approximately 3 Years and Above)

 9. ___

 10. ___

 11. ___

 12. ___

Electrophysiological Tests (Any Age)

 13. ___

 14. ___

 15. ___

 16. ___

Select From

A. Auditory brainstem response

B. Auropalpebral reflex

C. Acoustic reflex threshold

D. Behavioral observation audiometry

E. Conditioned orientation reflex

F. High-risk registry

G. Moro reflex

H. Noisemakers

I. Operant conditioning audiometry

J. Otoacoustic emissions

K. Play audiometry

L. Speech recognition threshold

M. Tympanometry

N. Visual response audiometry

O. Warblet

P. Word-recognition tests

MULTIPLE CHOICE

  1. The six sounds of the Ling six-sound test are
     a. aa (as in back), f, s, j, r, and v
     b. oo (as in move), ee (as in beet), ah (as in father), sh, s, and m
     c. oo (as in book), i (as in kick), aa (as in back), f, r, and th
     d. f, s, sh, t, k, and m

  2. Probably the easiest nonlanguage child to misdiagnose is the one with a hearing loss in
     a. the low frequencies
     b. the high frequencies
     c. the speech frequencies
     d. all frequencies

  3. Difficulties encountered when using noisemakers to test neonates is control of
     a. distance
     b. intensity
     c. frequency
     d. all of the above

  4. The "eye blink response" from infants to loud sounds is called
     a. ABR
     b. COR
     c. Moro reflex
     d. APR

  5. Minimum sensory deprivation syndrome may be suspected of children with
     a. repeated otitis media
     b. Rh incompatibility
     c. family history of hearing loss
     d. prematurity

  6. Present evolution of neonatal screening recommends that it should be performed
     a. on all neonates
     b. on neonates failing one part of the high-risk register
     c. on neonates who seem not to hear
     d. on no neonates

7. Electrodermal audiometry has been largely abandoned as a test for small children because
   a. the stimuli are too noxious for most children
   b. results were often unreliable
   c. further habilitation efforts are often affected adversely because of the child's fears
   d. all of the above

8. COR utilizes
   a. one loudspeaker and one lighted doll
   b. one loudspeaker and two lighted dolls
   c. two loudspeakers and one lighted doll
   d. two loudspeakers and two lighted dolls

9. ABR has some limits in pediatric diagnosis because
   a. it does not provide information about hearing in the low frequencies
   b. it does not provide information about hearing in the high frequencies
   c. it provides information only about the speech frequencies
   d. none of the above

10. Normal speech-detection thresholds in children do not necessarily mean normal hearing because
    a. hearing may be normal only in the low- or high-frequency range
    b. the SRT may be poorer than the SDT
    c. both a and b
    d. none of the above

11. An infant's startle response to a loud sound may mean
    a. normal hearing in both ears
    b. normal hearing in one ear
    c. a moderate hearing loss with recruitment
    d. all of the above

12. Ideally, public school hearing screening programs would include
    a. pure-tone screening
    b. pure-tone screening and tympanometry
    c. pure-tone screening, tympanometry, and acoustic reflexes
    d. pure-tone screening, tympanometry, acoustic reflexes, and SRTs

13. In operant conditioning the reinforcer should
    a. immediately follow the response
    b. be tangible
    c. be positive
    d. all of the above

14. Otoacoustic emissions have an advantage in neonatal hearing testing in that they
    a. are stable and reliable
    b. can be measured when the child is asleep or awake
    c. are unaffected by medications used to put a child to sleep
    d. all the above

VOCABULARY

auditory brainstem response (ABR)
auropalpebral reflex (APR)
behavioral observation audiometry (BOA)
conditioned orientation reflex (COR)
crib-o-gram
high-risk registry
Moro reflex
operant conditioning audiometry (OCA)
otoacoustic emission
pediacoumeter
peep show
play audiometry
respiration audiometry
visual reinforcement audiometry (VRA)

ANSWERS

Matching	*Outline*	*Multiple Choice*
1. d	**1.** B	**1.** b
2. j	**2.** F	**2.** b
3. b	**3.** O	**3.** d
4. e	**4.** D	**4.** d
5. h	**5.** G	**5.** a
6. l	**6.** E	**6.** a
7. i	**7.** H	**7.** d
8. c	**8.** N	**8.** d
9. k	**9.** I	**9.** a
10. g	**10.** K	**10.** a
11. a	**11.** L	**11.** d
12. f	**12.** P	**12.** c
	13. A	**13.** d
	14. C	**14.** d
	15. J	
	16. M	

THE INNER EAR

BACKGROUND

Since the animal brain cannot utilize sound vibrations, the function of the cochlea of the inner ear is to transduce the mechanical energy delivered from the middle ear into a form of energy that can be interpreted by the brain. The cochlea is a snail-shaped structure that is contained within the petrous portion of the temporal bone, the hardest bone in the body. The outer shell is called the bony labyrinth and contains a fluid called perilymph. Within the bony labyrinth is the membranous labyrinth, which is about one-third the size of the bony labyrinth and contains a slightly different fluid called endolymph.

Three ducts, called scalae, are arranged within the cochlea. The scala vestibuli is found just beyond the oval window and travels the length of the cochlea to a tiny hole at its apex called the helicotrema. Perilymph passes through the helicotrema to the scala tympani, which ends at the round window. From the perspective of the middle ear, the oval and round windows move 180 degrees out of phase as the incompressible perilymph moves to and fro.

Between the scala vestibuli and the scala tympani lies a third duct called, logically, the scala media, or cochlear duct, which contains endolymph. The scala media is separated from the scala vestibuli by Reissner's membrane and from the scala tympani by the basilar membrane. The basilar membrane supports the organ of Corti, which is the end organ for hearing. Impulses are sent from the cochlea to the brain in a bioelectrical code.

Damage to the cochlea produces the type of hearing loss known as sensorineural. In most cases, with some dramatic exceptions, cochlear hearing losses are irreversible and can occur at any age, in one or both ears, and can range from slight to profound. In addition to the loss of loudness, patients with cochlear hearing loss usually report difficulties in the discrimination of speech that may also vary in degree. For this reason measurements of speech recognition are essential if these cases are to be managed properly (see Unit 19).

In addition to information about hearing, the inner ear also reports to the brain impulses related to the body's position and movement. Like the cochlea, the balance, or vestibular portion of the inner ear, is comprised of a bony and membranous labyrinth. Two structures just within the inner ear are the end organs that interpret linear acceleration—that is, the movement of the head in a straight line. These structures are the utricle and the saccule. In addition, three loops called the semicircular canals provide information about angular acceleration of the head's rotation. Faulty information from the vestibular portion of the inner ear produces the sometimes-debilitating symptom of vertigo. Like the cochlea, the vestibular structures send information to the balance-interpreting portions of the brain by a neuroelectrical code.

In summary, the inner ear is called a labyrinth, which is Greek for a series of winding passages. Although extremely tiny, it is a myriad of hydromechanical and neuroelectrical activity. Through the cochlea the inner ear converts the mechanical acoustical vibrations of the middle ear into a form of energy, which the brain ultimately perceives as sound. Damage to the cochlea causes hearing losses that are termed sensorineural. Cochlear hearing losses result from a wide variety of causes and can occur at any age. Through its vestibular apparatus the inner ear provides the brain with the sensation of the head's position and motion in space. Proper testing of the vestibular mechanism has restored patients to a normal life when appropriate treatment is instituted.

OBJECTIVES

1. You should know and understand the terms in the matching exercise.

2. You should be able to fill in the outline, selecting items from the list provided.

3. You should be able to label the different parts of the inner ear as shown in Figures 8.1 and 8.2.

4. You should be able to answer the multiple-choice questions and understand the anatomy and physiology of the inner ear as well as the causes of disorders that produce sensorineural hearing loss in the inner ear.

5. You should know and understand the terms in the vocabulary list and be able to describe or define each term.

MATCHING

Match the term from the column on the right with its definition.

Definition

1. ___   The efferent portion of a neuron

2. ___   A procedure designed to monitor spontaneous or induced nystagmus

3. ___   Fluid contained in the vestibular and cochlear portions of the bony labyrinth that surrounds the membranous labyrinth

4. ___   The central portion of a nerve cell

5. ___   A vascular strip along the outer wall of the scala media that supplies oxygen to the cochlea

6. ___   The cavity of the inner ear that contains the organs of equilibrium

7. ___   Nerves that carry impulses from the periphery to the brain

8. ___   Three loops within the vestibule that monitor angular acceleration

9. ___   The smaller of two sacs in the vestibule that is responsible for sensing linear acceleration

10. ___   The cochlear duct containing the organ of Corti

11. ___   The widened ends of the semi-circular canals that contain the cristae

12. ___   Oscillatory movement of the eyes

13. ___   Fluid contained in the membranous labyrinth

14. ___   The membrane separating the scala media from the scala tympani and supporting the organ of Corti

15. ___ The interconnecting canals in the temporal bone

16. ___ The branching portion of a neuron that carries impulses to the cell body

17. ___ The duct in the inner ear above the scala media that contains perilymph

18. ___ The larger of two sacs in the vestibule that is responsible for sensing linear acceleration

19. ___ Nerves that carry impulses from the brain to the periphery

20. ___ The sensation of true turning or spinning

21. ___ The membrane separating the scala vestibuli from the scala media

22. ___ The membrane in the scala media above the organ of Corti into which the tips of the outer hair cells are embedded

23. ___ The duct below the scala media that is filled with perilymph

24. ___ An opening at the apical end of the cochlea connecting the scala vestibuli with the scala tympani

25. ___ A cell specialized for conveying nerve impulses

26. ___ A cavity in the temporal bone containing the end organ of hearing

Term

a. Afferent

b. Ampulla

c. Axon

d. Basilar membrane

e. Cell body

f. Cochlea

g. Dendrite

h. Efferent

i. Electronystagmography

j. Endolymph

k. Helicotrema

l. Labyrinth

m. Neuron

n. Nystagmus

o. Perilymph

p. Reissner's membrane

q. Saccule

r. Scala media

s. Scala tympani

t. Scala vestibuli

u. Semicircular canals

v. Stria vascularis

w. Tectorial membrane

x. Utricle

y. Vertigo

z. Vestibule

OUTLINE

The Inner Ear

Anatomy of the Cochlea

1. ___
2. ___
3. ___
4. ___
5. ___
6. ___
7. ___
8. ___
9. ___
10. ___
11. ___
12. ___
13. ___

Anatomy of the Vestibule

14. ___
15. ___
16. ___
17. ___
18. ___
19. ___

Disorders

20. ___
21. ___
22. ___
23. ___
24. ___
25. ___
26. ___
27. ___
28. ___

Select from

A.   Ampulla
B.   Anoxia
C.   Basilar membrane
D.   Cortilymph
E.   Crista
F.   Drug-induced
G.   Ductus reuniens
H.   Hair cells
I.   Helicotrema
J.   Macula
K.   Ménière disease
L.   Noise-induced
M.   Organ of Corti
N.   Otosclerosis
O.   Prenatal viral infections
P.   Presbycusis
Q.   Postnatal viral infections
R.   Reissner's membrane
S.   Saccule
T.   Scala media
U.   Scala tympani
V.   Scala vestibuli
W.   Semicircular canals
X.   Skull fracture
Y.   Spiral ligament
Z.   Stria vascularis
AA.   Tectorial membrane
AB.   Utricle

ACTIVITIES

Label the parts of the labyrinth and cross section of the cochlea in the figures that follow. Select the names from the lists provided.

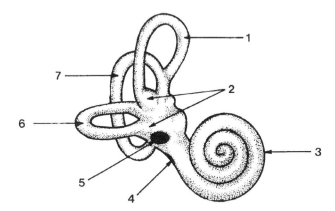

FIGURE 8.1   The labyrinth

Label	*Term*
1. ___	**A.** Ampullae
2. ___	**B.** Cochlea
3. ___	**C.** Horizontal (lateral) semicircular canal
4. ___	**D.** Inferior (posterior) semicircular canal
5. ___	**E.** Oval window
6. ___	**F.** Round window
7. ___	**G.** Superior (anterior) semicircular canal

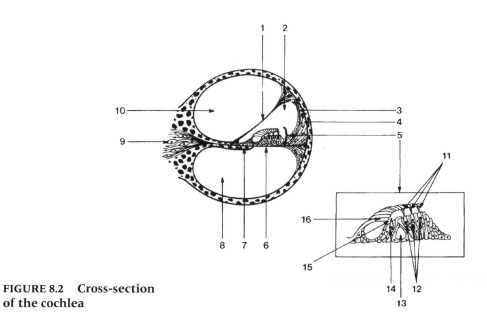

FIGURE 8.2   Cross-section of the cochlea

Label	*Term*
1. ___	**A.** Basilar membrane
2. ___	**B.** Inner hair cell cilia
3. ___	**C.** Inner hair cells
4. ___	**D.** Organ of Corti
5. ___	**E.** Outer hair cell cilia
6. ___	**F.** Outer hair cells
7. ___	**G.** Reissner's membrane
8. ___	**H.** Scala media (endolymph)
9. ___	**I.** Scala tympani (perilymph)
10. ___	**J.** Scala vestibuli (perilymph)
11. ___	**K.** Spiral ganglion
12. ___	**L.** Spiral lamina
13. ___	**M.** Spiral ligament
14. ___	**N.** Stria vascularis
15. ___	**O.** Tectorial membrane
16. ___	**P.** Tunnel of Corti

MULTIPLE CHOICE

1. A device used to measure oscillatory movement of the eyes in response to caloric stimulation is called an
   a. electronystagmograph
   b. electroencephalograph
   c. electromyograph
   d. audiograph

2. The stria vascularis does not
   a. carry blood
   b. support hair cells
   c. produce a DC potential
   d. produce endolymph

3. The type of cerebral palsy most associated with cochlear hearing loss is
   a. spasticity
   b. rigidity
   c. athetosis
   d. ataxia

4. Angular acceleration is measured in
   a. cm/sec^2
   b. cm/sec
   c. degrees/sec
   d. $degrees/sec^2$

5. The macula is the end organ located within the
   a. semicircular canals
   b. cochlea
   c. utricle
   d. brain

6. _____ does not make up a wall of the cochlear duct
   a. bony shelf
   b. tectorial membrane
   c. basilar membrane
   d. Reissner's membrane

7. Endolymph is found in the
   a. tectorial membrane
   b. scala vestibuli
   c. scala media
   d. scala tympani

8. The fluid surrounding the membranous labyrinth is called
   a. cortilymph
   b. perilymph
   c. endolymph
   d. lymph

9. The portion of the inner ear that responds to angular acceleration is called
   a. macula
   b. semicircular canals
   c. organ of Corti
   d. utricle

10. The central core around which the cochlea winds is the
    a. modiolus
    b. Reissner's membrane
    c. helicotrema
    d. basilar membrane

11. The tips of the outer hair cells are embedded in
    a. Reissner's membrane
    b. the bony shelf
    c. the tectorial membrane
    d. the basilar membrane

12. The most common postnatal cause of bilateral hearing loss from viral infection is
    a. rubeola (measles)
    b. rubella (German measles)
    c. pertussis (whooping cough)
    d. varicella (chicken pox)

13. Linear acceleration is measured in
    a. cm/sec^2
    b. cm/sec
    c. degrees/sec
    d. $degrees/sec^2$

14. Which of the following is not considered a perinatal cause of hearing loss?
    a. anoxia
    b. trauma
    c. rubella
    d. prolonged labor

15. Deprivation of oxygen, which may cause damage to the cochlea (and the brain), is called
    a. dysphemia
    b. dyscalculia
    c. dyslogia
    d. anoxia

16. The small opening allowing passage of perilymph from scala vestibuli to scala tympani is called
    a. modiolus
    b. stria vascularis
    c. spiral ligament
    d. helicotrema

17. The number of turns of the cochlea is
    a. 2
    b. $2\frac{1}{2}$
    c. 3
    d. $3\frac{1}{2}$

18. The structure just medial to the oval window is the
    a. cochlea
    b. semicircular canals
    c. vestibule
    d. helix

19. The crista is the end organ of the
    a. utricle
    b. saccule
    c. cochlea
    d. semicircular canals

20. Rapid back and forth movement of the eyes is called
    a. vertigo
    b. nystagmus
    c. dizziness
    d. near sightedness

21. The fluid contained in the membranous labyrinth is
    a. perilymph
    b. cortilymph
    c. blood
    d. endolymph

22. The end organ of hearing is the
    a. crista
    b. macula
    c. helicotrema
    d. organ of Corti

23. The portion of the inner ear responsible for linear acceleration is the
    a. semicircular canals
    b. utricle and saccule
    c. crista
    d. organ of Corti

24. During caloric testing when a normal left ear is stimulated with cold water, the eye beat is
    a. right
    b. left
    c. random
    d. unpredictable

25. Endolymph differs from perilymph because in endolymph
    a. potassium concentration is greater
    b. potassium concentration is less
    c. sodium concentration is greater
    d. resting microvoltage is less

26. Screening for hearing loss in the ultra-high-frequency range is often useful in detecting hearing loss caused by
    a. noise
    b. infection
    c. Ménière disease
    d. ototoxic drugs

27. Ménière disease is associated with
    a. bilateral hearing loss, good speech recognition
    b. unilateral hearing loss, poor speech recognition
    c. unilateral hearing loss, good speech recognition
    d. normal vestibular findings

28. Hereditary cochlear hearing loss resulting from genetic and environmental interactions is called
    a. homozygous
    b. hereditodegenerative
    c. multifactorial
    d. x-linked

29. Rh interactions put a baby at risk when
   a. mother is positive, father is positive
   b. mother is negative, father is negative
   c. mother is positive, father is negative
   d. mother is negative, father is positive

30. Presbycusis is hearing loss associated with
   a. aging
   b. noise
   c. bacterial infection
   d. viral infection

31. Sudden unilateral cochlear hearing loss may be caused by
   a. spasm of the internal auditory artery
   b. Ménière disease
   c. labyrinthitis
   d. all of the above

32. A hearing loss due to aging that is associated with loss of outer hair cells and supporting cells in the basal turn of the cochlea is called
   a. sensory presbycusis
   b. neural presbycusis
   c. strial presbycusis
   d. cochlear conductive presbycusis

33. Associated with cochlear hearing loss is
   a. loudness decruitment
   b. excellent speech discrimination
   c. loudness recruitment
   d. usual eligibility for surgical correction

34. The ABR latency-intensity function for wave V expected in cochlear hearing losses is
   a. increased, primarily at high intensities
   b. increased, primarily at low intensities
   c. decreased, primarily at high intensities
   d. decreased, primarily at low intensities

VOCABULARY

action potential

afferent

ampulla

axon

basilar membrane

cell body

cochlea

dendrite

ductus reuniens

efferent

electronystagmography (ENG)

endolymph

helicotrema

labyrinth

neuron

nystagmus

organ of Corti

perilymph

Reissner's membrane

saccule

scala media

scala tympani

scala vestibuli

semicircular canals

stria vascularis

tectorial membrane

utricle

vertigo

vestibule

ANSWERS

Matching	*Outline*	*Activities*
1. c	**1.** C	Figure 8.1 Labyrinth
2. i	**2.** D	**1.** G
3. o	**3.** G	**2.** A
4. e	**4.** H	**3.** B
5. v	**5.** I	**4.** F
6. z	**6.** M	**5.** E
7. a	**7.** R	**6.** C
8. u	**8.** T	**7.** D
9. q	**9.** U	Figure 8.2 Cross-section of cochlea
10. r	**10.** V	**1.** G
11. b	**11.** Y	**2.** H
12. n	**12.** Z	**3.** N
13. j	**13.** AA	**4.** M
14. d	**14.** A	**5.** D
15. l	**15.** E	**6.** A
16. g	**16.** J	**7.** L
17. t	**17.** S	**8.** I
18. x	**18.** W	**9.** K
19. h	**19.** AB	**10.** J
20. y	**20.** B	**11.** E
21. p	**21.** F	**12.** F
22. w	**22.** K	**13.** P
23. s	**23.** L	**14.** C
24. k	**24.** N	**15.** B
25. m	**25.** O	**16.** O
26. f	**26.** P	
	27. Q	
	28. X	

Multiple Choice

1. a		**18.** c
2. b		**19.** d
3. c		**20.** b
4. d		**21.** d
5. c		**22.** d
6. b		**23.** b
7. c		**24.** a
8. b		**25.** a
9. b		**26.** d
10. a		**27.** b
11. c		**28.** c
12. a		**29.** d
13. a		**30.** a
14. c		**31.** d
15. d		**32.** a
16. d		**33.** c
17. b		**34.** b

MASKING FOR
PURE-TONE TESTS

BACKGROUND

Surveys and personal observation lead to the inescapable conclusion that no single audiological procedure is as controversial and shows more divergent approaches than clinical masking. It is not known why this is the case, but despite some excellent methods for the accurate and scientific execution of masking, in many cases masking is not performed properly.

Masking may be defined as the elevation of the threshold of a stimulus produced by a second, concurrent stimulus. The sound that is masked is called the signal, and the sound that elevates the threshold is called the masker. In pure-tone audiometry the signal is a pure tone and the masker is a noise. Probably what confuses clinicians most about masking is the notion, acquired early in their education and training, that masking takes place with a signal in one ear and a masker in the other ear. This is because that is what the clinician DOES, but it is not what really happens. Actually, for a signal to be masked, the masker must also be heard in the same ear. Perhaps an analogy to vision can be helpful in understanding this very important concept. When taking a vision test, everyone knows that one eye is covered (masked) while the other eye is tested. This allows the examiner to know which eye is being examined. If one wants to keep visual images from being picked up by the right eye, it does little good to cover the left eye. There is a strong parallel to auditory masking.

We need to mask when we fear that a signal, like a pure tone, presented to one ear (say the right ear) is actually being heard in the opposite (left) ear because the signal has crossed the skull. Therefore, if the sound in this illustration is being heard in the left ear (by contralateralization), it is the left ear that must be masked. If the signal presented to the right ear has not reached the left ear, presentation of an effective level of noise to the left ear will have no effect on the audibility of the tone.

A masking noise should be specified in terms of its spectrum and its efficiency in producing a threshold shift. Unless audiologists understand the effectiveness of the masking noise they use, they can do little more than work in the dark. Clinical masking must be applied whenever there is a danger that a signal presented to the test ear may reach the threshold of the nontest ear by cross hearing. Cross hearing for air conduction (AC) signals is generally considered to occur primarily by bone conduction (BC). What happens is that at high intensities supra-aural earphones will actually be set into mechanical vibration and distort the skull in the same way that a bone-conduction oscillator does. Since insert receivers utilize a soft sponge placed in the external ear canal instead of a hard-rubber cushion pressed against the ear as used with supra-aural receivers, it takes much more energy for the vibration of the receiver to be transferred to vibration of the skull. When the skull is vibrated, the cochlea with lower bone-conduction thresholds is the one that will perceive the signal, whether that cochlea is on the same or opposite side of the head as the earphone.

The loss of intensity of a signal as it travels from the test ear air-conduction earphone to the cochlea of the nontest ear is called interaural attenuation (IA). IA averages from 50 to 65 dB for supra-aural receivers and from 70 to 100 dB for insert receivers. IA varies with different people and with frequency but has not been reported to be less than 40 dB for supra-aural phones or 70 dB for inserts. These are conservative values to use when deciding on the need to mask.

Since BC oscillations stimulate both cochleas with essentially equal force, the IA for BC is considered to be 0 dB. Therefore, interaural attenuation cannot be a part of the determination of whether masking is necessary during bone-conduction tests as it is for air conduction. Since it is normally not possible to know which cochlea responds during bone-conduction tests, some clinicians mask for bone-conduction tests in every case. This is done as a prudent approach to avoid cross hearing but results in time and energy being spent unnecessarily in many instances. Masking for bone conduction must be implemented when it might make a difference in diagnosis—that is, when there is an air-bone gap (ABG) in the test ear greater than 10 dB. If cross hearing has taken place for either air conduction or bone conduction, the only way the threshold of the test ear can be determined is by the plateau method. Because the masking noise to be used during bone-conduction testing is delivered through an air-conduction receiver, there is a chance that the masked ear may experience the occlusion effect. It is possible to assess the amount of the occlusion effect by performing the audiometric Bing test. After that is done, the occlusion effect (not usually seen at frequencies above 1000 Hz) must be added to the effective masking level as determined for air conduction. Failure to take this last step may result in undermasking for bone conduction. Just as the clinician must determine if a test signal is of sufficient intensity to be heard in the opposite ear, so must he or she be aware of when a masking signal presented to the nontest ear may be of sufficient intensity to cross the skull and cause masking in the test ear. The same IA values apply for considerations of cross hearing of the signal as one would use for consideration of potential cross hearing of the masker.

On commercial clinical audiometers the reference levels for masking pure tones with narrow noise bands, as specified by the American National Standards Institute (ANSI), are close to the values for pure tone thresholds in sound pressure level (SPL). The reference SPL for speech noise is approximately 20 dB SPL, the same as it is for speech. Zero decibels on the masking hearing level dial therefore tells the clinician nothing about the effect of the masking noise on the threshold of pure-tone and speech signals and how much additional noise is required to barely mask out a signal at different intensities. The concept of effective masking (EM) for clinical testing is very practical and easy to use once the audiometer has been properly calibrated or, more usually, corrections for calibration are made. Effective masking may be defined as the amount of threshold shift provided by a given level of noise. Thus, 20 dB EM at 1000 Hz is just enough noise to make a 20 dB HL 1000 Hz tone inaudible; 50 dB EM would just mask out a 50 dB HL tone, and so on. In the presence of 50 dB EM, a tone will not become audible until it reaches approximately 55 dB HL, regardless of an individual's hearing loss (assuming the hearing loss is less than 55 dB). This is true because any hearing loss attenuates both the tone and the masking noise equally. Since audiometers do not arrive with the masking circuits calibrated in effective masking, calibration is necessary to generate correction factors, and clinicians must remember that whenever they desire a given effective masking level, the correction factor must be added.

In most clinics calibration of effective masking is carried out psychoacoustically. Using about a dozen normal-hearing subjects, calibration may be accomplished as follows:

1. Present a 1000 Hz tone at 30 dB HL to one ear by air conduction. The tone is pulsed on and off to prevent auditory fatigue.

2. Present a noise (preferably narrowband) to the same ear. A second audiometer channel must be used.

3. Raise the level of the noise in 5 dB steps until the 30 dB tone is no longer audible. The tone should be heard again at about 35 dB HL. Recheck several times for accuracy.

4. Take a mean value for your dozen normal-hearing subjects of the masking-level dial setting at which the 30 dB HL tone was just barely masked.

5. Add 10 dB as a safety factor to offset the normal dispersion found around any mean. This is 30 dB EM at 1000 Hz.

6. Repeat this procedure for all audiometric frequencies.

7. Subtract 30 dB from the above value. This is 0 dB EM.

8. Post a correction chart on the audiometer showing the number of decibels that must be added to the hearing level dial reading to reach 30 dB EM for that intensity for each frequency. That correction factor must be added every time masking is used and is applicable for signals at any intensity.

An example of how this works is shown on the following table (units are in decibels). Assume that the average for the dozen normal-hearing subjects shows that at 1000 Hz a 30 dB HL tone is barely masked with a 45 dB HL masking noise. Note that in the first and last columns the level of effective masking is the same as the signal to be masked, as long as the correction factor is added.

Hearing Level of tone	Hearing Level of Noise in Same Ear to Just Mask Out Tone	Difference	Safety Factor	Correction Factor to Be Applied	Masking Level Dial Reading for this Effective Masking Level	Effective Masking
30	45	15	10	+25	55	30
20	35	15	10	+25	45	20
10	25	15	10	+25	35	10
0	15	15	10	+25	25	0

Once calibration has been completed, any level at any frequency can be masked (in the same ear) up to the maximum masking limits of the audiometer simply by adding the determined correction factor to the threshold level of the ear to be masked. If, for example, a +25 dB correction is needed for 0 dB EM (as in the above example) and a 40 dB tone is to be masked, the masking-level dial should be set to 40 dB EM, which is actually 65 dB HL (40 dB for the tone to be masked plus a 25 dB correction, which includes the safety factor). The safety factor is therefore built into the correction, and it should not be added again when determining individual masking levels. Therefore, any level of effective masking is equal to the threshold of the signal plus the correction factor. Stated as a formula this reads:

EM = Threshold + Correction Factor

The maximum amount of masking that can be delivered will, of course, be the limit of the attenuator, usually 110 dB HL. The level of effective masking will be less than that, of course, and will equal the maximum output minus the correction factor. Thus, given a theoretical correction factor of 25 dB, if the dial extends to 110 dB HL, the maximum effective masking will be 85 dB EM (110 – 25).

Of course, when masking is done clinically, the masker is presented to the earphone opposite the test earphone. Using this procedure assumes that the test tone may have lateralized and is actually heard in the masked ear. Therefore, if the tone has indeed lateralized, introduction of an EM level equal to the threshold of the masked ear should render the tone inaudible. (This would be the threshold value of the masked ear plus the correction factor.) At this point, the masking plateau process may begin. If the tone has not lateralized, introduction of that same level of masking into the nontest ear will allow the tone to remain audible (as it is still being heard in the test ear), and the masking exercise is complete for the frequency tested.

After working with effective masking for a short period of time most clinicians think in those values, even though the hearing level dial reading required to deliver a given amount of effective masking will always be a higher intensity. Inclusion of the correction factor becomes second nature. If sufficient thought is given to when and how to mask, there is really no reason why it cannot be carried out precisely and relatively easily in most cases. This requires motivation on the part of the clinician and demands that this procedure be taken seriously. The alternative to proper masking is incorrect diagnosis, which can lead to serious consequences.

OBJECTIVES

1. You should know and understand the terms in the matching exercise.

2. You should be able to fill in the outline, selecting items from the list provided.

3. Based on the audiogram in Figure 9.1A, you should be able to determine the need to mask for each frequency for air conduction and bone conduction.

4. You should be able to determine the minimum amount of noise required to just mask out the nontest ear, when necessary.

5. You should be able to label the parts of the masking plateau model in Figure 9.2.

6. You should be able to answer the multiple-choice questions and grasp the fundamental concepts of masking.

7. You should know and understand the terms in the vocabulary list and be able to describe or define each term.

MATCHING

Match the term from the column on the right with its definition

Definition

1. ___   A broadband noise containing approximately equal energy per cycle

2. ___   The level of noise that can be varied over a small range that does not alter the threshold of a sound presented to the opposite ear

3. ___   Introduction of noise into the nontest ear to eliminate cross-hearing

4. ___   The hearing of a sound in the ear opposite the one being tested

5. ___   The loss of energy of a sound as it travels from the test ear to the nontest ear

6. ___   A slight shift in threshold of a signal produced by a signal presented to the opposite ear that is not caused by peripheral (crossed) masking

7. ___   A band of frequencies surrounding a pure tone that is just wide enough to produce a threshold shift

8. ___   Masking of a stimulus produced by a noise in the nontest ear that crosses the skull and shifts the threshold of the test ear

9. ___   The lowest level of effective masking presented to the nontest ear during audiometry

10. ___   A broadband masking noise with energy concentrated in the low frequencies

11. ___ A system for calibrating a masking signal for simple operation of clinical masking procedures

12. ___ A restricted band of frequencies surrounding a particular frequency to be masked

13. ___ The highest level of noise that can be presented to one ear before it crosses the skull and masks the opposite ear

14. ___ The result of insufficient noise presented to the nontest ear so that the threshold of the test ear cannot be determined

Term

a. Central masking

b. Complex noise

c. Critical band

d. Cross hearing

e. Effective masking

f. Initial masking

g. Interaural attenuation

h. Masking

i. Maximum masking

j. Narrowband noise

k. Overmasking

l. Plateau

m. Undermasking

n. White noise

OUTLINE

Masking for Pure Tones

The Need to Mask

For AC

  1. ___

For BC

  2. ___

  3. ___

Interaural Attenuation

For AC

  4. ___

For BC

  5. ___

The Plateau Components

  6. ___

  7. ___

  8. ___

  9. ___

  10. ___

Noise Types

  11. ___

  12. ___

  13. ___

  14. ___

  15. ___

Occlusion Effect—Frequencies

  16. ___

  17. ___

  18. ___

Select From

A. ABG greater than 10 dB in test ear

B. $AC_{TE} - IA \geq BC_{NTE}$

C. Average 55 dB (minimum 40 dB) for supra-aural receivers; average 85 dB (minimum 70 dB) for inserts

D. Broadband

E. Complex

F. In all cases

G. Maximum masking

H. Minimum masking

I. Narrowband

J. Overmasking

K. Pink

L. Plateau

M. Sawtooth

N. Undermasking

O. 0 dB

P. 250 Hz

Q. 500 Hz

R. 1000 Hz

ACTIVITIES

In Table 9.1 indicate in the proper box whether masking is needed for the audiogram in Figure 9.1 and the minimum amount of effective masking required to mask the nontest ear.

TABLE 9.1   Masking for an Audiogram

	TONE RIGHT (MASKING LEFT)			
	AC		BC	
Frequency (Hz)	Masking Needed?	Min EM	Masking Needed?	Min EM
250		20		20 + OE
500		35		35 + OE
1000		45		45 + OE
2000		—		40
4000		—		—
	TONE LEFT (MASKING RIGHT)			
250		—		50 + OE
500		—		55 + OE
1000		—		55 + OE
2000		—		—
4000		—		—

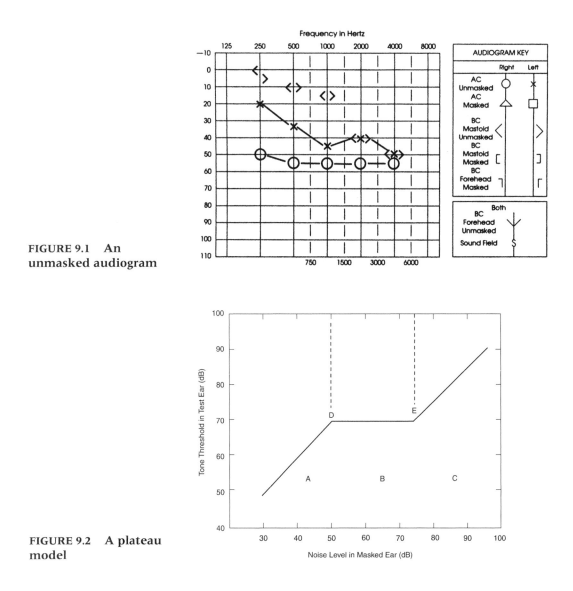

FIGURE 9.1 An unmasked audiogram

FIGURE 9.2 A plateau model

Label the five components of the plateau model.

1. _____

2. _____

3. _____

4. _____

5. _____

MULTIPLE CHOICE

1. Cross hearing is a possibility during pure-tone air conduction tests when
   a. $SRT_{TE} - 35$ dB $= BC_{NTE}$
   b. $ABG > 10$ dB
   c. $AC_{TE} - IA \geq BC_{NTE}$
   d. $AC_{TE} - BC_{NTE} = ABG$

2. The primary way by which cross hearing for air conduction takes place is by
   a. skin conduction
   b. air conduction
   c. bone conduction
   d. cartilage conduction

3. The energy lost as sound travels from one ear to the other is called
   a. interaural attenuation
   b. cross-hearing
   c. contralateralization
   d. lateralization

4. The occlusion effect is tested during the ___ test.
   a. Bing
   b. Rinne
   c. Schwabach
   d. Weber

5. Minimum masking for bone conduction at 250 Hz is
   a. $EM = AC_{TE} + OE$
   b. $EM = AC_{NTE} + OE$
   c. $EM = AC_{TE} - IA$
   d. $EM = AC_{NTE} - IA$

6. Unmasked results on a patient with one normal ear and one ear with a total sensorineural loss show the poorer ear to have
   a. moderate conductive hearing loss
   b. moderate sensorineural hearing loss
   c. profound conductive hearing loss
   d. normal hearing

7. The audiometric Bing test determines the need for additional masking for
   a. bone conduction
   b. word recognition
   c. air conduction
   d. SRT

8. A predicted loss of sensitivity to an auditory stimulus in the presence of contralateral noise is called
   a. overmasking
   b. undermasking
   c. initial masking
   d. central masking

9. Masking is indicated for bone conduction when
   a. $ABG_{TE} > 10$ dB
   b. $ABG_{NTE} > 10$ dB
   c. $BC_{TE} - BC_{NTE} > 10$ dB
   d. $AC > 40$ dB

10. Overmasking is the greatest problem in
    a. bilateral conductive loss
    b. unilateral conductive loss
    c. bilateral sensorineural loss
    d. unilateral sensorineural loss

11. The most efficient kind of masking noise for pure-tone testing is
    a. narrowband noise
    b. broadband noise
    c. high-pass filtered noise
    d. pink noise

12. The masking plateau becomes narrower as the
    a. BC threshold in the test ear gets lower (better)
    b. BC threshold in the test ear gets higher (poorer)
    c. interaural attenuation gets greater
    d. AC threshold in the test ear gets lower (better)

13. As the interaural attenuation increases, the masking plateau
    a. stays the same
    b. gets narrower
    c. gets wider
    d. changes in midfrequencies

14. Overmasking takes place for air conduction when
    a. $BC_{TE} + IA = EM_{NTE}$
    b. $BC_{TE} + IA - 10$ dB $= EM_{NTE}$
    c. $EM_{NTE} - ABG_{NTE} <$ True AC_{TE}
    d. $EM_{NTE} - ABG_{NTE} =$ True AC_{TE}

VOCABULARY

air-bone gap (ABG)	minimum masking
cross hearing	minimum masking for normals
effective masking (EM)	nontest ear (NTE)
insert receiver	occlusion effect (OE)
interaural attenuation (IA)	overmasking (OM)
masker	plateau
masking	test ear (TE)
maximum masking	undermasking

ANSWERS

Matching	*Outline*	*Multiple Choice*
1. n	**1.** B	**1.** c
2. l	**2.** A	**2.** c
3. h	**3.** F	**3.** a
4. d	**4.** C	**4.** a
5. g	**5.** O	**5.** b
6. a	**6.** G	**6.** a
7. c	**7.** H	**7.** a
8. k	**8.** J	**8.** d
9. f	**9.** L	**9.** a
10. b	**10.** N	**10.** a
11. e	**11.** D	**11.** a
12. j	**12.** E	**12.** a
13. i	**13.** I	**13.** c
14. m	**14.** K	**14.** a
	15. M	
	16. P	
	17. Q	
	18. R	

Activities

TABLE 9.2   Masking for an Audiogram (answers)

	TONE RIGHT (MASKING LEFT)			
	AC		**BC**	
Frequency (Hz)	Masking Needed?	Min EM	Masking Needed?	Min EM
250	yes	20	yes	20 + OE
500	yes	35	yes	35 + OE
1000	yes	45	yes	45 + OE
2000	no	—	yes	40
4000	no	—	no	—
	TONE LEFT (MASKING RIGHT)			
250	no	—	yes	50 + OE
500	no	—	yes	55 + OE
1000	no	—	yes	55 + OE
2000	no	—	no	—
4000	no	—	no	—

Figure 9.2   Plateau Model

1. Undermasking

2. Plateau (range of EM in decibels)

3. Overmasking

4. Minimum masking

5. Maximum masking

■ ■ ■ ■ ■ ■ ▬▬▬▬▬▬▬▬▬▬▬▬▬▬▬▬▬▬▬▬▬▬▬▬▬▬▬

MASKING FOR SPEECH TESTS

BACKGROUND

The challenge of detecting the need for and proper use of masking for speech audiometry is, in many ways, similar to masking for pure tones (Unit 9). The possibility of cross hearing during pure-tone tests is determined by comparing the air-conduction (AC) threshold of the test ear (TE) to the bone-conduction (BC) threshold of the nontest ear (NTE) at the same frequency. This is done frequency by frequency. If the difference exceeds what may be the interaural attenuation (IA) for a given frequency, retesting must be done with masking in the nontest ear. The old procedure of looking for a "good ear" and "bad ear" is often a misleading approach.

Because it should be assumed that cross hearing occurs by bone conduction, the determination of whether a speech signal has been cross heard is slightly more complicated than it is for pure tones because the level of this complex broadband signal (speech), presented by air conduction to one ear, must be compared to a pure-tone threshold obtained by bone conduction in the opposite ear. Since it cannot be known which of the frequencies in the nontest ear may contribute to the cross hearing of a speech signal, it is safest to compare to the lowest (best) bone-conduction threshold at 500, 1000, 2000, or 4000 Hz; frequencies below 500 Hz contribute very little to the discrimination of speech. When the interaural difference equals or exceeds a conservative figure set for interaural attenuation (40 dB for supra-aural earphones, 70 dB for insert earphones), cross hearing may have occurred and masking should be applied to the nontest ear to render it temporarily incapable of responding. Stated as a formula:

Need to Mask for SRT

$$SRT_{TE} - IA => Lowest\ BC_{NTE}$$

Forty decibels is substituted for IA in the formula when supra-aural earphones are used and 70 dB is substituted when insert earphones are used.

Masking is most efficiently carried out if the masking noise is calibrated in decibels of effective masking (EM) for speech. To do this the steps outlined in Unit 9 should be followed substituting "SRT" for "Hearing Level of Tone." The noise spectrum should be broader than the narrowbands used for pure-tone masking and is usually called "white noise," "broadband noise," or "speech noise." The problem of overmasking is greatest during SRT testing when there is a hearing loss in the masked ear (requiring a higher level of noise) and an air-bone gap (ABG) in the test ear. This is because the more intense masker may lateralize to the test ear by bone conduction and raise its threshold.

Any level of effective masking is the hearing-level dial setting for the SRT plus the correction factor. For example, given a correction factor of +25 dB, to find 0 dB EM (the amount of noise that will be required to mask a 0 dB SRT) the hearing-level dial is set to 25 dB HL, 50 dB EM has a dial setting of 75 dB HL, and so forth. This is identical to the pure-tone approach. That should be just enough to prevent the nontest ear from responding. If the initial effective masking level results in the second SRT being unchanged from the first, it may be assumed that the unmasked SRT is correct and no further masking is required for SRT for that ear. If, with the nontest ear just masked out, the patient does not repeat any of the spondees, it must be assumed that the original SRT was obtained by cross hearing and the masking plateau must be sought. The best way to proceed is to obtain all thresholds initially with no masking, even if it is obvious from the outset of testing that masking will be required. After that is done, the audiologist can examine the pure-tone thresholds by air and bone conduction and the SRTs to determine whether masking is indicated for any of these tests.

The need to mask to determine speech recognition scores (SRS) is more complicated than just described for SRT because speech-recognition tests are suprathreshold rather than threshold tests. These tests are usually done 30 or 40 dB above the SRT and often at much higher levels, like 90 dB HL. After SRTs are obtained, either with or without masking, the hearing level of the speech-recognition test is chosen. That level may be called the PBHL when phonetically balanced word lists are used, and it is then compared to the lowest bone-conduction threshold of the nontest ear. Again, stated as a formula this reads:

Need to Mask to Determine Speech-Recognition Scores

$PBHL_{TE} => Lowest\ BC_{NTE}$

The method determining the amount of masking required in the administration of SRSs is likewise more complicated. The simplest way to do this is to follow this formula:

Effective Masking Level Needed to Determine Speech-Recognition Scores

$EM = PBHL_{TE} - IA + (largest)\ ABG_{NTE}$

The air-bone gap must be added, if one exists, because it (the conductive component of the hearing loss) attenuates the masking noise that leaves the masking earphone before it reaches the cochlea. Since the effective masking level is always higher for tests that measure the SRS than it is for those that measure the SRT, the possibility of overmasking is greater in the former case. Many times masking is required when determining the SRS when it is not needed to find the SRT. This accentuates the advantages of using insert receivers, which increase the interaural attenuation of the speech signal from the test ear to the nontest ear (by at least 30 dB), as well as increasing the interaural attenuation of the noise from the masked ear to the test ear (by at least another 30 dB). This provides an additional interaural separation of at least 60 dB, significantly cutting down the odds of overmasking. The problem of overmasking is greatest during speech-recognition testing when there is an air-bone gap in the masked ear and fairly good bone conduction in the test ear.

Masking is sometimes used during speech tests like most-comfortable loudness (MCL) and uncomfortable loudness (UCL), but this appears to be unusual. Adherence to the principles just described for SRT and SRS tests can be applied to these other measures.

Failure to recognize the need to mask during speech audiometry, or to carry out masking properly, carries with it the same dangers of misdiagnosis as it does for pure-tone testing. It is probable that clinicians who ignore the rules described above for speech audiometry do likewise for pure-tone audiometry. The result is that the goal of having speech audiometry serve as a reliability check for pure-tone audiometry is not accomplished. Consequences for this can be significant for the patient.

OBJECTIVES

1. You should know and understand the terms in the matching exercise.

2. You should be able to fill in the outline, selecting items from the list provided.

3. You should be able to determine the need to mask, based on an audiogram and unmasked SRTs.

4. You should be able to determine the minimum amount of effective masking noise required to just mask out the nontest ear when necessary.

5. You should be able to determine when overmasking has taken place.

6. You should be able to answer the multiple-choice questions and grasp the fundamental concepts of masking for speech audiometry.

7. You should know and understand the terms in the vocabulary list and be able to describe or define each term.

MATCHING

Match the term from the column on the right with its definition.

Definition

1. ___ The ear opposite the one being tested

2. ___ The loss of energy of a (speech) sound as it travels from one ear to the other

3. ___ The lowest intensity at which approximately 50 percent of a list of spondees can be identified correctly

4. ___ The difference (in decibels) between the air-conduction and bone-conduction thresholds in the same ear

5. ___ Insufficient noise to eliminate the nontest ear from participation in a speech test

6. ___ The greatest amount of noise that can be delivered to the nontest ear without overmasking

7. ___ The act of the nontest ear hearing a speech signal that is presented to the test ear

8. ___ A noise level high enough to lateralize from the nontest ear to the test ear and shift the threshold of the test ear

9. ___ The percentage of correctly identified items on a word-recognition test

10. ___ The least amount of noise required to barely mask out a signal in the same ear

11. ___ The ear being examined on a hearing test

Term

a. Air-bone gap

b. Cross hearing

c. Effective masking

d. Interaural attenuation

e. Masking

f. Maximum masking

g. Minimum masking

h. Nontest ear

i. Overmasking

j. PB hearing level

k. Plateau

l. Speech-recognition threshold

m. Test ear

n. Undermasking

o. Word-recognition score

12. ___ The intensity at which a noise in the nontest ear can be elevated three times without affecting the audibility of a speech signal in the test ear

13. ___ A reasonable system for calibration of a masking noise

14. ___ The elevation of the threshold of a signal produced by the introduction of a second signal

15. ___ The hearing level at which an audiometer is set to carry out word-recognition testing with PB word lists

OUTLINE

Masking for Speech Tests

The Need to Mask

For SRT

  1. ___

For SRS

  2. ___

Interaural Attenuation

  3. ___

  4. ___

Minimum EM for SRT

  5. ___

Minimum EM for SRS

  6. ___

Noise Type

  7. ___

Select From

A. Average 55 dB for supra-aural phones, 90 dB for insert phones

B. Broadband

C. Equal to SRT of NTE

D. Minimum 40 dB for supra-aural phones, 70 dB for insert phones

E. $PBHL_{TE} - IA + ABG_{NTE}$

F. $PBHL_{TE} - IA \geq$ lowest BC_{NTE}

G. $SRT_{TE} - IA \geq$ lowest BC_{NTE} (not including 250 Hz)

ACTIVITIES

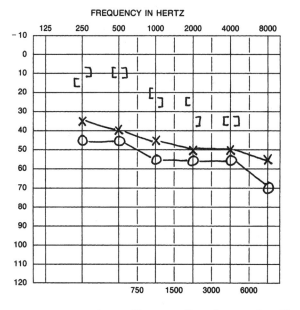

FIGURE 10.1   An audiogram showing a mixed loss in both ears

In Table 10.1 indicate in the proper box whether masking is needed for SRT and speech-recognition testing for each ear; also indicate the minimum amount of effective masking required to mask the nontest ear (if necessary). Assume that the speech-recognition test is done at 35 dB above the SRT and supra-aural earphones are used.

TABLE 10.1   Chart for Masking

	SPEECH RIGHT (MASKING LEFT)			SPEECH LEFT (MASKING RIGHT)		
Test	*Masking Needed?*	*Minimum EM*	*Test*	*Masking Needed?*	*Minimum EM*
SRT 55 dB			SRT 45 dB		
SRS ? %			SRS ? %		

MULTIPLE CHOICE

1. Of the following the most efficient masker to use during speech audiometry is
   a. narrowband noise
   b. broadband noise
   c. pure tone
   d. the identical signal presented to the test ear

2. It is always necessary to mask for speech-recognition testing when
   a. there is an air-bone gap in the test ear greater than 25 dB
   b. the patient's interaural attenuation exceeds 30 dB
   c. the audiograms are asymmetrical
   d. masking was needed for SRT testing

3. The interaural attenuation for speech can be determined if
   a. there is an air-bone gap in the test ear
   b. the unmasked SRT is obtained by cross hearing
   c. the test ear has a conductive hearing loss
   d. the test ear has a sensorineural hearing loss

4. For speech-recognition tests, overmasking creates the greatest problem in
   a. bilateral mixed loss
   b. unilateral mixed loss
   c. bilateral sensorineural loss
   d. unilateral sensorineural loss

5. The need to mask during SRT testing is determined by comparing the
   a. SRT of the test ear to the pure-tone average of the nontest ear
   b. SRT of the test ear to the SRT of the nontest ear
   c. unmasked SRT to the opposite ear bone-conduction thresholds
   d. SRT of the test ear to the interaural attenuation

6. The need to mask during speech-recognition testing is determined by comparing the
   a. hearing level of the test stimuli (PBHL) to the opposite ear bone-conduction thresholds
   b. SRT of the test ear to the interaural attenuation
   c. SRT of the test ear to the SRT of the nontest ear
   d. none of the above

7. Overmasking occurs during SRT testing when the
   a. test presentation level exceeds 95 dB
   b. interaural attenuation is greater than 60 dB
   c. test presentation level exceeds the SRT of the nontest ear
   d. effective masking level minus the patient's interaural attenuation equals or exceeds the bone-conduction thresholds of the test ear

8. Overmasking occurs during speech-recognition testing when the
   a. test presentation level exceeds 95 dB
   b. interaural attenuation is greater than 60 dB
   c. test presentation level exceeds the SRT of the nontest ear
   d. effective masking level minus the patient's interaural attenuation meets or exceeds the bone-conduction thresholds of the test ear

9. The result of not masking, when required during speech-recognition threshold testing, may be that the
   a. SRT was obtained by bone conduction in the nontest ear
   b. SRT was obtained by air conduction in the nontest ear
   c. SRT was actually lower (better) than what was observed
   d. none of the above

10. The result of not masking, when required during speech-recognition testing, may be that the
    a. speech-recognition score is actually poorer than that which is observed
    b. nontest ear actually took the speech-recognition test
    c. speech-recognition test was actually taken by both ears
    d. all of the above

11. The result of overmasking during speech-recognition threshold testing may be that the
    a. SRT appears better than it truly is
    b. SRT appears worse than it truly is
    c. interaural attenuation is increased
    d. none of the above

12. The result of overmasking during speech-recognition testing may be that the
    a. speech-recognition score appears better than it truly is
    b. speech-recognition score appears poorer than it truly is
    c. sensation level of the test is raised
    d. none of the above

13. When a patient's interaural attenuation is not known, it is safest to assume that it may be as little as _____ dB when testing with insert receivers
    a. 30
    b. 70
    c. 50
    d. 60

14. The air-bone gap of the masked ear must be added to minimum masking levels during speech-recognition testing because
    a. the conductive component of the loss attenuates the masking level
    b. the interaural attenuation is increased in conductive hearing losses
    c. masking is always needed when the test ear has a conductive hearing loss
    d. none of the above

15. Five decibels is often added to the usual sensation level for speech-recognition tests when masking is used to
    a. increase the interaural attenuation
    b. decrease the interaural attenuation
    c. account for cross hearing
    d. offset central masking

16. If the interaural attenuation for speech can be determined to be greater than 40 dB when supra-aural earphones are used, it is better to use the larger number to
    a. increase the likelihood of undermasking
    b. decrease the likelihood of undermasking
    c. decrease the likelihood of overmasking
    d. increase the likelihood of overmasking

17. Overmasking during SRT testing results in the
    a. SRT of the nontest ear getting higher (poorer)
    b. SRT of the nontest ear getting lower (better)
    c. SRT of the test ear getting higher (poorer)
    d. SRT of the test ear getting lower (better)

18. One excellent means of minimizing the chances of undermasking or overmasking during speech audiometry is to
    a. test with insert receivers
    b. mask with insert receivers
    c. test and mask with insert receivers
    d. use supra-aural earphones

VOCABULARY

air-bone gap (ABG)
cross hearing
effective masking (EM)
insert receiver
interaural attenuation (IA)
masking
maximum masking
minimum masking

nontest ear (NTE)
overmasking (OM)
PB hearing level (PBHL)
plateau
speech-recognition score (SRS)
speech-recognition threshold (SRT)
test ear (TE)
undermasking

ANSWERS

Matching

1. h
2. d
3. l
4. a
5. n
6. f
7. b
8. i
9. o
10. g
11. m
12. k
13. c
14. e
15. j

Outline

1. G
2. F
3. A
4. D
5. C
6. E
7. B

Activities

TABLE 10.2   Chart for Masking

	SPEECH RIGHT (MASKING LEFT)			SPEECH LEFT (MASKING RIGHT)		
Test	*Masking Needed?*	*Minimum EM*	*Test*	*Masking Needed?*	*Minimum EM*
SRT 55 dB	yes	45 dB	SRT 45 dB	no	—
SRS ? %	yes	80 dB	SRS ? %	yes	75 dB

Multiple Choice

1. b		**10.** d	
2. d		**11.** b	
3. b		**12.** b	
4. a		**13.** b	
5. c		**14.** a	
6. a		**15.** d	
7. d		**16.** c	
8. d		**17.** c	
9. a		**18.** c	

THE MIDDLE EAR

BACKGROUND

The middle ear is a tiny air-filled space designed to match the impedance of air in the outer ear canal to the impedance of fluid in the inner ear. There is, of course, a middle ear on each side of the head. Because the middle ear is in the conductive portion of the auditory system, abnormalities in this region affect a patient's air-conduction threshold with minimal effects on bone conduction. When only the middle ear is involved, a hearing loss should be purely conductive and may range from very mild to moderately severe. Air-bone gaps greater than 60 dB are quite rare (see Unit 18). If both the middle ear and inner ear are disordered, either from common or unrelated causes, a mixed hearing loss will be present. Damage to the middle ear and other portions of the auditory system are not mutually exclusive. Dysfunction of the middle ear may result from disease, trauma, or hereditary conditions.

The middle ear carries vibrations from the outer ear to the inner ear by transferring the sound energy from the air in the outer ear to the fluids of the inner ear by two basic mechanisms. First, the vibrating area of an average tympanic membrane is about 55 mm^2, which is approximately seventeen times the area of the oval window. Pressure collected over the surface of the tympanic membrane is therefore increased by concentrating it over this much smaller area; much like water pressure leaving a garden hose can be increased by holding a thumb over the opening. Since sound energy is carried from the tympanic membrane, which separates the outer ear from the middle ear, along a chain of three tiny bones (the ossicles) to the oval window, which separates the middle ear from the inner ear, the sound pressure is naturally increased. In this way the middle ear overcomes the loss of energy that results when sound passes from one medium (in this case, air in the outer ear canal) to another medium (fluid in the inner ear).

An understanding of the basics of hearing tests is valuable in understanding the implications of middle-ear disorders. Abnormalities of the structure or function of the middle ear result in conductive hearing losses, wherein the air-conduction thresholds are depressed in direct relationship with the amount of disease or abnormality. Bone-conduction thresholds may deviate slightly from normal in conductive hearing losses, not because of abnormality of the sensorineural mechanism, but because of alterations in the middle ear's normal (inertial) contribution to bone conduction (see Unit 4).

Alterations in pressure-compliance functions give general information regarding the presence of fluid or negative air pressure in the middle ear, stiffness, or interruption of the ossicular chain. Measurements of static compliance may be higher or lower than normal, and acoustic reflex thresholds are either elevated or absent (see Unit 14). Auditory brain stem responses show increased latencies for all waves and otoacoustic emissions are usually absent (see Unit 14). Results on speech-recognition tests are the same as for those with normal hearing (see Unit 19).

Middle-ear hearing loss can come about because of perforation of the tympanic membrane, loss or stiffening of the ossicular chain, fluid accumulation in the middle-ear space because of disease or structural abnormality, as well as many other causes. Treatment for disorders of the middle ear is best administered by an otolaryngologist (a specialist in ear, nose, and throat [ENT]). Remediation of middle-ear disorders should first be concerned with medical or surgical reversal of the problems. When this fails, must be postponed, or is not available, careful audiological counseling should be undertaken, and treatment avenues, such as the use of hearing aids, preferential seating in the classroom, and educational supplementation should be investigated. Provided there are no medical contraindications to hearing aid use and no planned medical or surgical intervention, patients with conductive hearing losses are excellent candidates for hearing aids because of their relatively flat audiometric contours, good speech recognition, and tolerance for loud sounds.

OBJECTIVES

1. You should know and understand the terms in the matching exercise.

2. You should be able to fill in the outline, selecting items from the list provided.

3. You should be able to label the different parts of the middle ear shown in Figure 10.1.

4. You should be able to answer the multiple-choice questions and understand the anatomy and physiology of the middle ear as well as the causes of disorders that produce conductive hearing loss.

5. You should know and understand the terms in the vocabulary list and be able to describe or define each term.

MATCHING

Match the term from the column on the right with its definition.

Definition

1. ___ The largest of the ossicles, which is attached to the tympanic membrane

2. ___ An operation to reverse hearing loss caused by otosclerosis, carried out by breaking the stapes footplate free

3. ___ An artifact in bone conduction in patients with otosclerosis

4. ___ A surgical procedure to restore middle-ear function

5. ___ The VIIth cranial nerve

6. ___ The second bone in the ossicular chain that connects the malleus to the stapes

7. ___ The chain of three tiny bones in the middle ear

8. ___ Sterile fluid accumulation in the middle ear

9. ___ An operation to remove infection from the mastoid

10. ___ A space in the superior portion of the middle-ear space

11. ___ The Vth cranial nerve

12. ___ A small muscle that can impede movement of the malleus

13. ___ Inflammation of the mastoid

14. ___ An operation designed to improve hearing loss caused by otosclerosis by removing the stapes and replacing it with a prosthesis

15. ___ The attic of the middle-ear space

16. ___ The moist lining of the middle-ear space

17. ___ Infection of the middle ear

18. ___ In anatomy, a leg, as of the stapes

19. ___ Formation of spongy bone that may affect the normal movement of the stapes

20. ___ Incision into the tympanic membrane, usually to remove fluid

21. ___ A membrane separating the middle ear from the inner ear

22. ___ A channel connecting the middle ear to the nasopharynx

23. ___ Calcium formations between layers of the tympanic membrane or in the middle ear, often caused by infection

24. ___ The smallest of the ossicles, which stands in the oval window

25. ___ An older operation to correct hearing loss from otosclerosis

26. ___ A membrane, supporting the footplate of the stapes, that separates the middle ear from the inner ear

27. ___ A small muscle, connected to the stapes, that impedes movement of the ossicles when it is contracted

28. ___ A collection of fats and other debris in the middle ear, usually caused by infection

Term

a. Aditus ad antrum

b. Carhart notch

c. Cholesteatoma

d. Crus

e. Epitympanic recess

f. Eustachian tube

g. Facial nerve

h. Fenestration

i. Incus

j. Malleus

k. Mastoidectomy

l. Mastoiditis

m. Mucous membrane

n. Myringotomy

o. Ossicles

p. Otitis media

q. Otosclerosis

r. Oval window

s. Round window

t. Serous effusion

u. Stapedectomy

v. Stapedius muscle

w. Stapes

x. Stapes mobilization

y. Tensor tympani muscle

z. Trigeminal nerve

aa. Tympanoplasty

ab. Tympanosclerosis

OUTLINE

The Middle Ear

Anatomy

1. ___
2. ___
3. ___
4. ___
5. ___
6. ___
7. ___

Bones

8. ___
9. ___
10. ___

Muscles

11. ___
12. ___

Disorders

13. ___
14. ___
15. ___
16. ___
17. ___
18. ___

Surgical Treatment

19. ___
20. ___
21. ___
22. ___
23. ___
24. ___

Select From

A. Aditus ad antrum
B. Congenital abnormalities
C. Epitympanic recess
D. Eustachian tube
E. Fenestration
F. Fractures
G. Incus
H. Malleus
I. Mastoidectomy
J. Middle-ear space
K. Myringotomy
L. Otitis media
M. Otosclerosis
N. Oval window
O. Round window
P. Serous effusion
Q. Stapedectomy
R. Stapes
S. Stapes mobilization
T. Stapedius
U. Tensor tympani
V. Tympanic membrane
W. Tympanoplasty
X. Tympanosclerosis

ACTIVITY

Select the terms from the list provided and label the parts of the middle ear in Figure 11.1

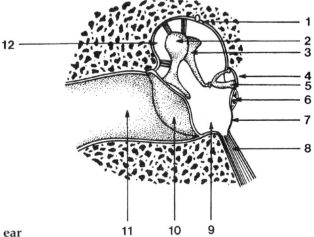

FIGURE 11.1   The middle ear

Label		*Term*
1. ___		**A.** Aditus ad antrum
2. ___		**B.** Epitympanic recess
3. ___		**C.** Eustachian tube
4. ___		**D.** External auditory canal
5. ___		**E.** Incus
6. ___		**F.** Malleus
7. ___		**G.** Middle-ear space
8. ___		**H.** Oval window
9. ___		**I.** Promontory
10. ___		**J.** Round window
11. ___		**K.** Stapes
12. ___		**L.** Tympanic membrane

MULTIPLE CHOICE

1. The chain of bones in the middle ear is called the
   a. malleus
   b. incus
   c. stapes
   d. ossicles

2. Stapedectomy and stapedotomy have replaced stapes mobilization because
   a. there is less possibility of refixation
   b. the potential air-bone gap is small
   c. the operation is tolerated better
   d. they are less dangerous to perform

3. The general classification of surgical procedures for repairing damage of middle ear structures is
   a. tympanoplasty
   b. stapedialplasty
   c. rhinoplasty
   d. otoplasty

4. A pseudotumor in the middle ear composed of skin and fatty tissue is called
   a. otitis externa
   b. otosclerosis
   c. otitis media
   d. cholesteatoma

5. Which of the following is not a usual treatment for serous effusion?
   a. pressure-equalizing tubes
   b. mastoidectomy
   c. myringotomy
   d. decongestant medication

6. Pressure-equalizing tubes are designed to function primarily as an artificial
   a. ear canal
   b. mastoid
   c. eustachian tube
   d. hairpiece

7. The most popular surgical treatment for otosclerosis is
   a. fenestration
   b. tympanoplasty
   c. stapedotomy
   d. stapes mobilization

8. The manubrium is part of the
   a. malleus
   b. incus
   c. stapes
   d. eustachian tube

9. The eustachian tube connects the middle ear with the
   a. outer ear
   b. inner ear
   c. nasopharynx
   d. nose

10. Nonbacterial otitis media usually results from
   a. a blocked eustachian tube
   b. nasopharyngitis
   c. otitis media
   d. otosclerosis

11. Otosclerosis is
   a. equally common in men and women
   b. most common in men
   c. most common in women
   d. most common in children

12. Fluid in the middle-ear space may result from
   a. a blocked eustachian tube
   b. infection entering the middle ear via the eustachian tube
   c. infection entering the middle ear via the bloodstream
   d. all of the above

13. Hearing speech better in a noisy place than in a quiet place is a symptom of
   a. normal hearing
   b. conductive hearing loss
   c. sensorineural hearing loss
   d. none of the above

14. The Carhart notch is usually associated with
   a. otosclerosis
   b. bacterial otitis media
   c. serous effusion
   d. a blocked eustachian tube

15. Given a moderate conductive hearing loss in the right ear and normal hearing in the left ear, otoacoustic emissions are expected to be
   a. absent in both ear
   b. present in both ears
   c. present in the right ear, absent in the left ear
   d. present in the left ear, absent in the right ear

VOCABULARY

aditus ad antrum (tympanic aditus)

Carhart notch

cholesteatoma

conductive hearing loss

crus

epitympanic recess

Eustachian tube

facial nerve

fenestration

incus

malleus

mastoidectomy

mastoiditis

middle-ear space

mucous membrane

myringotomy

ossicles

otitis media

otosclerosis

oval window

round window

serous effusion (secretory otitis media)

stapedectomy

stapedius muscle

stapes

stapes mobilization

tensor tympani muscle

trigeminal nerve

tympanoplasty

tympanosclerosis

ANSWERS

Matching	Outline	Activity	Multiple Choice
1. j	**1.** A	**1.** A	**1.** d
2. x	**2.** C	**2.** F	**2.** a
3. b	**3.** D	**3.** E	**3.** a
4. aa	**4.** J	**4.** H	**4.** d
5. g	**5.** N	**5.** K	**5.** b
6. i	**6.** O	**6.** I	**6.** c
7. o	**7.** V	**7.** J	**7.** c
8. t	**8.** G	**8.** C	**8.** a
9. k	**9.** H	**9.** G	**9.** c
10. e	**10.** R	**10.** L	**10.** a
11. z	**11.** T	**11.** D	**11.** c
12. y	**12.** U	**12.** B	**12.** d
13. l	**13.** B		**13.** b
14. u	**14.** F		**14.** a
15. a	**15.** L		**15.** d
16. m	**16.** M		
17. p	**17.** P		
18. d	**18.** X		
19. q	**19.** E		
20. n	**20.** I		
21. s	**21.** K		
22. f	**22.** Q		
23. ab	**23.** S		
24. w	**24.** W		
25. h			
26. r			
27. v			
28. c			

NONORGANIC HEARING LOSS

BACKGROUND

Some patients seen for hearing evaluations may feign or exaggerate a hearing loss. Terms that have been used to describe this behavior include nonorganic hearing loss, pseudohypacusis, malingering, psychogenic hearing loss, functional hearing loss, conversion deafness, and a host of others. It is the responsibility of the audiologist to recognize nonorganic hearing loss and to determine the patient's true hearing status, albeit often without the patient's cooperation. Recognizing the presence of nonorganic hearing loss is usually not that difficult for an alert audiologist. Learning the true organic levels of hearing and finding a resolution to whatever the motivation may be are the real challenges.

There are numbers of reasons why an individual might decide to fabricate or exaggerate a disability, and many forms of expression for these decisions. Lawsuits have been filed for compensation for back pain, memory loss, cognitive deficits, spinal-cord injury, weakness, dizziness, and, of course, hearing loss. In addition, there is a host of litigious actions, many of which are related to claims for workers' compensation. Veterans of modern warfare are exposed to horrendous levels of noise that are known causes of hearing loss and the temptation to exaggerate a claim for VA benefits may be too much for some individuals to resist. Some children may express nonorganic hearing loss as a means of acquiring peer acceptance, parental affection, decreased academic pressures, and so on.

For some time the notion was that nonorganic hearing loss was either consciously feigned or motivated by some unconscious force. The term "malingering" describes the former group. This is a pejorative word indeed, for it implies out-and-out lying, something that is difficult or impossible to prove. The latter is a remnant of Freudian thinking and considers the possibility that some patients suffer from a form of conversion neurosis and that the symptom (in this case hearing loss) is merely a physical manifestation of a deep psychological disorder. In such "psychogenic" hearing losses, the patient is supposedly unaware of the falsification or exaggeration of a hearing loss. It is possible that there are bona fide examples of both these conditions, but it is also probable that most patients with nonorganic hearing loss can be found on a continuum between these two extremes. In most cases identification of etiology falls outside the purview of the audiologist.

The source of patient referral, medical history, symptoms, and behavior both during and outside of formal hearing tests are factors to be considered before making a diagnosis of nonorganic hearing loss. Observation of the patient and special tests for nonorganic hearing loss often lead the audiologist to the proper resolution of the problem. The responsibility of the audiologist is to determine the true organic thresholds of hearing, even if this must be done with less than the full cooperation of the patient.

The usual tip-off to a nonorganic hearing loss is inconsistency in test results. This may take the form of poor test-retest reliability, as when a threshold varies by more than 10 dB when it is remeasured. Or there may be poor intertest reliability, the classical example of which is a discrepancy between the SRT and the pure-tone average.

A number of tests can be performed when nonorganic hearing loss is suspected. Some of them merely confuse patients and provide evidence of nonorganicity; they might also convince the patients that they must be more cooperative. Included on this list are procedures like the Lombard test, delayed speech feedback, Variable Intensity Story test, and so on. Other tests, such as auditory evoked potentials and otoacoustic emissions, actually help determine auditory thresholds with a minimum of patient cooperation. Some other measures come close to identifying threshold but have limited utility, like the Stenger test, which is only suitable for unilateral hearing losses.

After diagnosis comes the usually more formidable task of patient management and, when indicated, appropriate referral. Audiologists have an obligation to serve patients even when they are uncooperative. The problems of writing reports and counseling are much greater with patients with nonorganic hearing loss than with those showing no evidence of this condition.

OBJECTIVES

1. You should know and understand the terms in the matching exercise.

2. You should be able to fill in the outline, selecting items from the list provided.

3. You should know which tests are appropriate for different kinds and degrees of nonorganic hearing loss.

4. You should know the equipment that is required for different tests for nonorganic hearing loss.

5. You should be able to answer the multiple-choice questions on nonorganic hearing loss.

6. You should know and understand the terms in the vocabulary list and be able to describe or define each term.

MATCHING

Match the term from the column on the right with its definition.

Definition

1. ___ A test for nonorganic hearing loss utilizing spondees and broadband noise

2. ___ The willful act of feigning a hearing loss or other disorder

3. ___ Early auditory evoked potentials

4. ___ Nonorganic hearing loss presumably at the unconscious level

5. ___ A test based on the fact that people speak more loudly when they hear a loud noise

6. ___ A term for claimed hearing loss that is not explainable in terms of organic pathology

7. ___ A synonym for nonorganic hearing loss

8. ___ A test for nonorganic hearing loss involving a delay between the time a patient taps a finger or utters a word and the time the sound is heard

Term

a. Auditory brain stem response

b. Delayed auditory feedback

c. Doerfler-Stewart test

d. Lombard test

e. Malingering

f. Nonorganic hearing loss

g. Pseudohypacusis

h. Psychogenic hearing loss

OUTLINE

Nonorganic Hearing Loss

Terminology

1. ____

2. ____

3. ____

4. ____

5. ____

6. ____

Test for Unilateral Nonorganic Hearing Loss

7. ____

General Tests for Nonorganic Hearing Loss

8. ____

9. ____

10. ____

11. ____

12. ____

Select From

A. Auditory brain stem response

B. Conversion deafness

C. Delayed auditory feedback

D. Doerfler-Stewart test

E. Functional hearing loss

F. Lombard test

G. Malingering

H. Nonorganic hearing loss

I. Pseudohypacusis

J. Psychogenic hearing loss

K. Stenger test

L. VIST

MULTIPLE CHOICE

1. When a nonorganic hearing loss is suspected, the audiologist may best increase cooperation by
   a. confronting the patient
   b. counseling the patient about his or her ethical responsibilities
   c. shifting the blame to the examiner
   d. insisting on greater attention to the tests

2. A nonorganic hearing loss of an unconscious nature is called
   a. sinistrosis
   b. psychogenic hearing loss
   c. nonorganic hearing loss
   d. malingering

3. The following is *not* an alerting sign for nonorganic hearing loss
   a. source of referral
   b. behavior during the interview/case history
   c. elevated acoustic reflexes
   d. performance on routine tests

4. The problem with most tests for nonorganic hearing loss is that they are
   a. nonqualitative
   b. nonquantitative
   c. too qualitative
   d. easy to beat

5. The following test for nonorganic hearing loss is limited to unilateral losses
   a. pure-tone delayed auditory feedback
   b. Stenger test
   c. Doerfler-Stewart test
   d. Lombard test

6. The following is a typical finding with nonorganic hearing loss
   a. SRT worse than PTA
   b. sensorineural loss with absent acoustic reflexes
   c. conductive loss with absent acoustic reflexes
   d. lack of cross hearing in unilateral loss

7. The Lombard test can be done as part of
   a. delayed-speech feedback
   b. Doerfler-Stewart test
   c. VIST
   d. Stenger test

8. In nonorganic hearing loss the general finding is
   a. SRT = PTA
   b. SRT lower (better) than PTA
   c. SRT higher (poorer) than PTA
   d. SRT = SDT

9. The following test gives the best estimate of threshold
   a. pure-tone DAF
   b. Stenger test
   c. Doerfler-Stewart test
   d. Lombard test

10. Elevation of vocal output in the presence of noise is called the
    a. Lombard voice reflex
    b. paracusis willisi
    c. Doerfler-Stewart effect
    d. Stenger effect

11. Malingering can be proven only if
    a. the patient admits it
    b. ABR reveals normal hearing
    c. the Stenger is positive
    d. otoacoustic emissions are present

12. Nonorganic hearing loss involving a deliberate act is called
    a. hysterical deafness
    b. psychogenic hearing loss
    c. nonorganic hearing loss
    d. malingering

13. Threshold can probably best be determined on a nonorganic hearing loss patient showing bilateral hearing loss with the
    a. VIST
    b. ABR
    c. Doerfler-Stewart test
    d. Stenger test

14. The minimum contralateral interference level is designed to
    a. screen for nonorganicity on the Stenger
    b. indicate precise threshold on the Stenger
    c. modify the Stenger
    d. approximate threshold on the Stenger

15. Key tapping is used with
    a. pure-tone DAF
    b. speech DAF
    c. LOCK test
    d. Békésy audiometry

16. The latest addition to the battery of tests for nonorganic hearing loss is
    a. otoacoustic emissions
    b. ABR
    c. Stenger test
    d. Lombard test

VOCABULARY

auditory brain stem response (ABR)
BADGE test
Békésy audiometry
delayed auditory feedback
Doerfler-Stewart (D-S) test
electrodermal audiometry (EDA)
functional hearing loss
galvanic skin response (GSR)
lengthened off time (LOT) test
Lombard test

malingering
nonorganic hearing loss
otoacoustic emission
pseudohypacusis
psychogenic hearing loss
Sensitivity Prediction from the
    Acoustic Reflex (SPAR)
Stenger test
swinging story test
Varying Intensity Story Test (VIST)

ANSWERS

Matching	Outline	Multiple Choice
1. c	**1.** B	**1.** c
2. e	**2.** E	**2.** b
3. a	**3.** G	**3.** c
4. h	**4.** H	**4.** b
5. d	**5.** I	**5.** b
6. f	**6.** J	**6.** d
7. g	**7.** K	**7.** a
8. b	**8.** A	**8.** b
	9. C	**9.** a
	10. D	**10.** a
	11. F	**11.** a
	12. L	**12.** d
		13. b
		14. d
		15. a
		16. a

NOISE

BACKGROUND

Some estimates show that for several years the level of noise in the environment increased by as much as a decibel a year. Since no noise in nature can threaten human hearing without being infinitely more dangerous to physical safety, it is humankind that has visited this modern epidemic upon itself. There is evidence that children are suffering increased amounts of hearing loss from such items as toy phones, musical instruments, firecrackers, stereo systems, and toy guns, some of which produce noise levels up to 155 dBA. Clearly, hearing awareness should be presented to school-age children as part of any Better Hearing and Speech Month activities.

Documented cases of noise-induced hearing loss go back more than 200 years. Hearing losses from intense noise may be the result of brief exposure to high-level sounds, with subsequent partial or complete hearing recovery, or repeated exposure to high-level sounds, with permanent impairment. Cases in which hearing thresholds improve after an initial impairment following noise are said to be the result of temporary threshold shift (TTS); irreversible losses are called permanent threshold shifts (PTS). In addition, a number of agents may interact with noise to increase the danger to hearing sensitivity. Research has shown that aspirin, which has been known to produce reversible hearing loss after ingestion, may synergize with noise to produce a greater temporary threshold shift than would otherwise be observed.

Acoustic trauma is the term often used to describe noise-induced hearing loss from impulsive sounds, such as explosions and gunfire, and audiometrically is frequently accompanied by an notch appearing between 3000 and 6000 Hz, with recovery at 8000 Hz, suggesting damage to the portion of the basal turn of the cochlea related to that frequency range. The Occupational Safety and Health Administration (OSHA) has recommended a scale on which the time that a worker may be safely exposed to intense sounds must be decreased as the intensity of the noise is increased. Under this rule, the maximum exposure level is 85 dBA (the A setting on a sound-level meter) for an eight-hour workday. For every 5 dB increase in noise, half the time is allowed—for example, four hours for 90 dBA, two hours for 95 dBA, one hour for 100 dBA, 30 minutes for 105 dBA, and so on. The National Institute of Occupational Safety and Health (NIOSH) has promulgated guidelines that for many audiologists are becoming the benchmark for standard of care. The NIOSH guidelines are more stringent than those set by OSHA in several areas, including noise monitoring, noise exposure limits, hearing monitoring practices, and the training of audiometric technicians. For example, NIOSH endorses a more protective 3 dB time-intensity tradeoff rather than OSHA's 5 dB exchange rate. Sound-level meters, or individually worn noise dosimeters, are used to measure the intensity of sound in noisy areas, such as in factories and around aircraft, to determine whether the noise levels fall within or exceed the damage-risk criteria set up by OSHA or recommended by NIOSH.

Many problems are associated with fitting and wearing hearing protectors, and the amount of sound attenuation found in the laboratory may be considerably more than that actually obtained on the job. It is likely that hearing protectors may provide a false sense of security, mistakenly assuring wearers that they are "safe" from noise damage. The more experience individuals have in inserting earplugs into their own ears, the greater the sound attenuation provided. Audiologists should warn hearing aid users that the hollow shell of a turned-off hearing aid provides little effective protection.

A surprising amount of the noise-induced hearing loss seen today is caused by other than work-related activities. Many millions of people are engaged in hobbies involving motorboats, snowmobiles, motorbikes, and race cars, in addition to the use of guns. The term "recreational audiology" has been coined to describe the activities of professionals involved in finding these hearing losses and helping those exposed to recreational noise to take appropriate precautionary steps. Exposure to intense sounds by professional musicians has caused a special concern for this group. Aerobic instructors and their students may be at particular risk from intense music exposure as studies have suggested that physical exercise plus noise results in greater threshold shifts than exposure to noise alone, possibly due to the effects on the cochlea of changes in metabolic activity during exercise. In addition to the auditory effects of intense noise, there is increasing evidence that noise may play a role in increased anxiety levels, loss of the ability to concentrate, higher divorce rates, greater incidence of illness, and loss of sleep.

Often, initial examination of hearing is made on the basis of a complaint of tinnitus alone. In patients with an acoustic trauma notch, the tinnitus is often described as a pure tone and can be matched to frequencies within the audiometric notch. Many of these patients are unaware of the existence of hearing loss and may even deny it. By the time progression of the impairment has been demonstrated to patients, their communicative difficulties may have worsened considerably. The persuasiveness and tact of the audiologist in counseling these patients is of paramount importance.

The audiologist should try to discover whether noise is a factor in a patient's hearing loss and then help, by counseling, to find ways of preventing progression of the loss. Many audiologists are active in the industrial, military, legal, and political arenas, where debates about noise continue to be waged.

OBJECTIVES

1. You should know and understand the terms in the matching exercise.

2. You should be able to fill in the outline, selecting items from the list provided.

3. You should know the factors in the environment that produce dangerous noise levels.

4. You should know some strategies for dealing with patients who are exposed to high noise levels, including counseling techniques and the fitting of hearing protectors.

5. You should be able to answer the multiple-choice questions on the subject of noise.

6. You should know and understand the terms in the vocabulary list and be able to describe or define each term.

MATCHING

Match the term from the column on the right with its definition

Definition

1. ___ Noise-induced hearing loss associated with sudden onset of intense noise

2. ___ A device that measures the intensity of noise over a period of time

3. ___ A federal agency designed to oversee the preservation of health and safety in the workplace

4. ___ Noise analysis with a sound-level meter that filters the sounds into narrowbands of one octave

5. ___ A reversible loss of hearing caused by intense noise

6. ___ Guidelines for avoiding noise-induced hearing loss that include noise intensity and time of exposure

7. ___ An irreversible loss of hearing caused by intense noise

8. ___ Any unwanted signal

Term

a. Acoustic trauma

b. Damage-risk criteria

c. Noise

d. Noise dosimeter

e. Octave-band analysis

f. OSHA

g. Permanent threshold shift

h. Temporary threshold shift

OUTLINE

Noise

Auditory Effects

   1. ___

   2. ___

   3. ___

   4. ___

   5. ___

Nonauditory Effects

   6. ___

   7. ___

   8. ___

   9. ___

Causes

  10. ___

  11. ___

  12. ___

Measurement

  13. ___

  14. ___

  15. ___

Damage-Risk Criteria

  16. ___

  17. ___

Agencies and Laws

  18. ___

  19. ___

  20. ___

  21. ___

Protection

  22. ___

  23. ___

Hearing Conservation

  24. ___

  25. ___

Select From

A. Acoustic trauma notch

B. Audiometric monitoring

C. EPA

D. Gunfire

E. Illness

F. Industry

G. Machinery

H. Muffs

I. Nervous disorders

J. NIOSH

K. Noise abatement

L. Noise dosimeter

M. Noise exposure time

N. Noise intensity

O. Noise survey

P. OSHA

Q. PTS

R. Plugs

S. Property damage

T. Psychological disorders

U. Sensorineural hearing loss

V. Speech interference

W. Sound-level meter

X. TTS

Y. Walsh-Healey Act

MULTIPLE CHOICE

1. The drop in high-frequency hearing sensitivity secondary to sudden noise exposure is often called
   a. anacusis
   b. Carhart notch
   c. otosclerosis
   d. acoustic trauma notch

2. An irreversible impairment of hearing secondary to intense noise exposure is called
   a. permanent threshold shift
   b. conductive hypacusis
   c. temporary threshold shift
   d. hypacusis

3. Many patients with noise-induced hearing loss report tinnitus in the frequency area of
   a. 250 Hz
   b. 500 Hz
   c. 4000 Hz
   d. 10,000 Hz

4. Sounds that produce a noise-induced hearing loss may be
   a. uncomfortably loud
   b. painful
   c. not uncomfortably loud
   d. all of the above

5. When the A scale of a sound-level meter is used, there is
   a. maximum deemphasis of the low frequencies
   b. moderate deemphasis of the high frequencies
   c. slight deemphasis of the high frequencies
   d. equal emphasis on all frequencies

6. Damage-risk criteria include the
   a. spectrum of the noise
   b. intensity of the noise
   c. duration of exposure
   d. all of the above

7. Maximum attenuation of noise is accomplished with
   a. acoustic earplugs in the ears
   b. fingers in the ears
   c. tragus pushed into the ear canal
   d. hands placed over the ears

8. Cases in which hearing thresholds improve after an initial impairment from excessive noise are called
   a. temporary threshold shift
   b. permanent threshold shift
   c. conductive hypacusis
   d. anacusis

9. The first federal act placing limits on noise levels allowable in workplaces doing government contract work was called
   a. ANSI
   b. ASA Act
   c. Walsh-Healey Act
   d. EPA Act

10. The filter setting used for most noise measurements on sound-level meters is the
    a. A scale
    b. B scale
    c. C scale
    d. D scale

11. Nonauditory effects of noise include
    a. property damage
    b. disease
    c. nervous conditions
    d. all of the above

12. A hunter who consistently fires a rifle from the right shoulder would be expected to have
    a. a greater loss in the right ear
    b. a greater loss in the left ear
    c. equal loss in both ears
    d. none of the above

VOCABULARY

damage-risk criteria
hearing protectors
Environmental Protection Agency (EPA)
forensic audiology
industrial audiology
National Institute for Occupational Safety
    and Health (NIOSH)
noise
noise dosimeter

noise-induced hearing loss
noise pollution
octave band analysis
Occupational Safety and Health
    Administration (OSHA)
permanent threshold shifts (PTS)
sound level meter (SLM)
temporary threshold shift (TTS)
Walsh-Healey Act

ANSWERS

Matching	*Outline*		*Multiple Choice*
1. a	1. A	14. O	1. d
2. d	2. Q	15. W	2. a
3. f	3. U	16. M	3. c
4. e	4. V	17. N	4. d
5. h	5. X	18. C	5. a
6. b	6. E	19. J	6. d
7. g	7. I	20. P	7. c
8. c	8. S	21. Y	8. a
	9. T	22. H	9. c
	10. D	23. R	10. a
	11. F	24. B	11. d
	12. G	25. K	12. b
	13. L		

OBJECTIVE TESTS
OF HEARING

BACKGROUND

While traditional audiological measures of pure-tone and speech audiometry require a patient's active cooperation, objective electroacoustical and electrophysiological procedures have been developed that require no behavioral responses from patients. These measures provide valuable information about hearing sensitivity and the site of lesion of an auditory disorder. Contemporary objective tests of hearing include immittance measures, which provide information about middle-ear status and the integrity of the neural pathways controlling the middle-ear muscles; auditory evoked responses, which measure the neuroelectric activity in the auditory system in response to sound; and the measure of transient acoustic signals emitted by the outer hair cells in the cochlea in response to sound stimulation.

The word immittance, when applied to measurements at the tympanic membrane, is a combined form of the words impedance (the opposition to the flow of acoustic energy to the middle ear) and admittance (that acoustic energy passed by the tympanic membrane into the middle ear). It is a compromise in terminology. Three major tests can be carried out with modern electroacoustic immittance meters: (1) static compliance—a means of determining the degree of stiffness of the tympanic membrane and ossicular chain; (2) tympanometry—a measure of the compliance of the tympanic membrane with varying degrees of positive and negative pressure in the external auditory canal; (3) the acoustic reflex threshold—determination of the intensity of a sound required to contract the stapedius muscle when that sound is presented to the same ear as the probe (ipsilateral acoustic reflex), which senses tympanic membrane movement, or to the opposite ear (contralateral acoustic reflex). Acoustic reflexes and the acoustic reflex decay test can help in determining the site of pathology in sensorineural losses, approximation of degree of hearing loss in noncooperative patients, facial nerve integrity, and more.

Acoustic immittance measurements give remarkably reliable information regarding the function of the middle ear. Both static compliance and tympanometry are measures of the mobility of the middle-ear mechanism. Distinctive tympanometric patterns, combined with audiometric findings, can aid the clinician in determining the underlying pathology of a conductive hearing loss. There is no doubt that the acoustic immittance meter has become as indispensable to the audiologist as the audiometer.

The auditory brain stem response (ABR) currently is used not only to estimate hearing sensitivity but also to help in determination of the site of auditory lesion. The development of averaging computers allows the presentation of numbers of stimuli so that the background activity in the brain can be averaged to near zero amplitude, while the series of wave peaks that signify responses at different points along the auditory pathway following stimulus introduction are increased in amplitude. All this serves to improve the signal-to-noise ratio with the signal being the neuroelectric response to a delivered sound and the noise being the normal ongoing neuroelectric activity of the brain. Responses are usually defined in terms of their latencies (time after stimulus onset), with the earliest responses occurring in the lower centers (e.g., the cochlea, auditory nerve, or brain stem) and the later responses in the auditory cortex.

Auditory brain stem response audiometry has become an important part of the site-of-lesion test battery, and some of the other evoked potential techniques are becoming more valuable as they are improved. Many of these tests have found their way into the operating room for monitoring during neurosurgery. Although the ABR should be considered to be more a test of synchronous neural firings than of hearing *per se*, its value to diagnostic audiology and to neurological screening is well established.

The realization that it was possible to measure weak sounds in the external auditory canal that could be evoked by transient acoustic signals led to the rapid clinical implementation of measures of otoacoustic emissions. This procedure, which is maturing at a remarkable rate, has the ability to screen the hearing of newborn infants in a brief and economical fashion and to contribute to the diagnosis of the site of lesion within the auditory system.

The introduction of otoacoustic emissions to the test battery is a giant leap in the direction of testing patients who cannot or will not cooperate during voluntary hearing tests. The advantages to using OAEs with children are obvious. This procedure is noninvasive and requires no patient cooperation, except to remain relatively motionless. Data-collection time has been estimated at 1 to 5 minutes per ear, which is very advantageous considering that children tend to be active. Otoacoustic emissions have added significantly to the battery of tests for site of lesion. OAEs may be used in combination with evoked potential measures to help differentiate sensory from neural lesions and may also be utilized as a crosscheck of middle-ear status, as determined by acoustic immittance measures.

The combination of acoustic immittance measures, auditory evoked potentials, and otoacoustic emissions has brought the profession of diagnostic audiology to an advanced status that could not have been predicted just a couple of decades ago. Over the life of the profession of audiology many exciting procedures have been introduced, greeted with great enthusiasm, and then found to be disappointing and abandoned. It is safe to predict that some form of the three procedures just described will be used by audiologists for many years to come.

OBJECTIVES

1. You should know and understand the terms in the matching exercise.

2. You should be able to fill in the outline, selecting items from the list provided.

3. You should understand the implications of static immittance, including its possible weaknesses as a measurement of true tympanic membrane function.

4. You should be able to interpret the different types of tympanograms, know how they are obtained, and what they imply.

5. You should know the implications of absent, elevated, and low sensation level acoustic reflex thresholds.

6. You should know some variations of the acoustic reflex test, including acoustic reflex decay, comparison of ipsilateral and contralateral acoustic reflex thresholds, and results of measurements made with different kinds of stimuli.

7. You should understand the different auditory evoked potential tests and what their latencies signify.

8. You should understand the principles of otoacoustic emission and the tests available.

9. You should be able to answer the multiple-choice questions on electrophysiological measurements.

10. You should know and understand the terms in the vocabulary list and be able to describe or define each term.

MATCHING

Match the term from the column on the right with its definition.

Definition

1. ___ The lowest intensity at which a stimulus produces an acoustic reflex

2. ___ The total contribution to impedance made by mass, stiffness, and frequency

3. ___ The VIIth cranial nerve, which runs from the brain stem to the stapedial tendon

4. ___ A small muscle whose insertion is in the neck of the stapes

5. ___ Measurement of the pressure-compliance function of the eardrum membrane

6. ___ Measurement of impedance or admittance of the eardrum membrane

7. ___ Contraction of the middle-ear muscles in response to sound

8. ___ A graph representing the pressure-compliance function of the eardrum membrane

9. ___ A small muscle whose insertion is in the neck of the malleus

10. ___ The inverse of stiffness

11. ___ That portion of impedance that is independent of frequency

12. ___ A unit of impedance measurement

13. ___ A decrease in the impedance of the eardrum membrane as a result of constant sound stimulation

14. ___ The ascending and descending pathways of the acoustic reflex

15. ___ Evoked potentials that appear 10 to 50 msec after signal onset (abbr.)

16. ___ Evoked potentials that appear 75 msec after signal onset with a large peak at a latency of 300 msec (abbr.)

17. ___ The third electrode used in auditory evoked potential testing that prevents the body from acting as an antenna

18. ___ The electrode used in auditory evoked potential testing that is unaffected by electrical activity in the brain

19. ___ Evoked potentials that appear within the first 10 msec after signal onset (abbr.)

20. ___ Evoked potentials that occur almost immediately after signal onset

21. ___ A graph drawn as a function of the delay in appearance of wave V versus the intensity required to produce the wave

22. ___ Evoked potentials that appear about 100 msec after signal onset (abbr.)

Term

a. ABR

b. Acoustic reflex

c. Acoustic reflex arc

d. AMLR

e. ART

f. Auditory event-related response

g. Compliance

h. ECochG

i. Facial nerve

j. Ground

k. Immittance

l. Latency-intensity

m. LER

n. Ohm

o. Reactance

p. Reference

q. Reflex decay

r. Resistance

s. Stapedius

t. Tensor tympani

u. Tympanogram

v. Tympanometry

OUTLINE

Electrophysiological Tests

Acoustic Immittance

Equipment

1. ___

2. ___

3. ___

4. ___

5. ___

6. ___

7. ___

8. ___

9. ___

Static Compliance

10. ___

11. ___

12. ___

13. ___

Tympanometry

14. ___

15. ___

16. ___

17. ___

18. ___

Acoustic Reflex

19. ___

20. ___

21. ___

22. ___

Select From

A. Absent—conductive or severe sensorineural loss

B. Air pump

C. Averaging computer

D. Balance meter

E. Clicks or tone bursts

F. Compliance with TM "loose"

G. Compliance with TM "tight"

H. Contralateral earphone

I. Elevated—mild conductive loss

J. Low value—stiffness of TM and/or ossicular chain

K. Loudspeaker

L. Low SL—cochlear lesion

M. High value—interruption of ossicular chain, flaccid TM

N. Manometer

O. Microphone

P. Oscillator

Q. Potentiometer

R. Probe assembly

S. Promontory electrodes and amplifier

T. Pure tone

U. Reflex decay—retrocochlear lesion

V. Scalp electrodes and amplifier

W. Type A—normal ME

X. Type B—fluid in ME

Y. Type C—negative pressure in ME

Z. Type A_S—stiffness of ossicular chain

Electrophysiological Tests

ABR

Stimulus

  23. ___

Equipment

  24. ___

  25. ___

Response Latency

  26. ___

ECochG

Stimulus

  27. ___

Equipment

  28. ___

  29. ___

Response Latency

  30. ___

LER

Stimulus

  31. ___

Equipment

  32. ___

  33. ___

Response Latency

  34. ___

AA. Type A_D—very compliant TM

AB. 8 msec or less

AC. 10 msec or less

AD. 50 to 300 msec

ACTIVITY

Sketch four different tympanograms on the following forms (Figures 14.1 to 14.4). Compare your graphs to the properly drawn tympanograms (Figures 14.5 to 14.8) at the end of this unit.

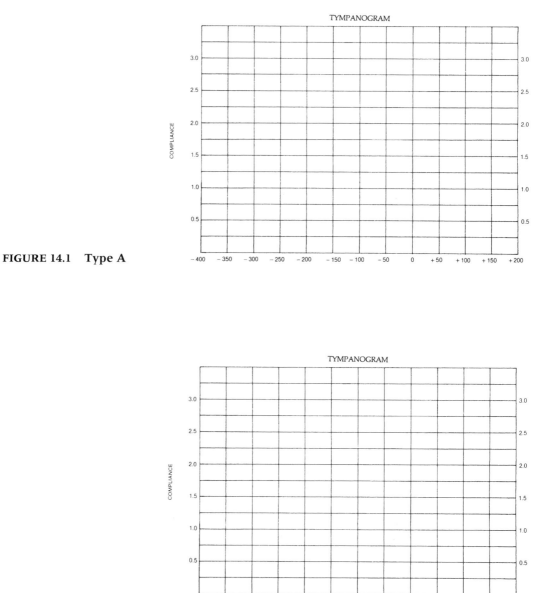

FIGURE 14.1 Type A

FIGURE 14.2 Type B

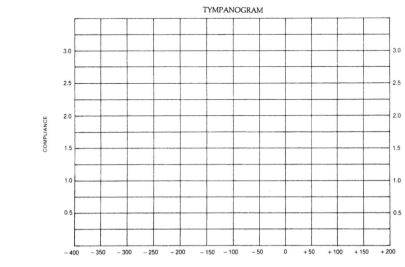

FIGURE 14.3   Type C

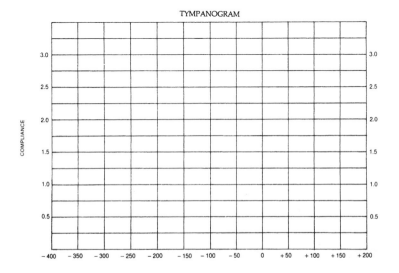

FIGURE 14.4   Type A$_S$

MULTIPLE CHOICE

1. Theoretically, a patient with otosclerosis should show
   a. normal tympanic membrane compliance
   b. higher than normal tympanic membrane compliance
   c. lower than normal tympanic membrane compliance
   d. fluctuating tympanic membrane compliance

2. Absence of an acoustic reflex is probable in
   a. conductive hearing loss
   b. profound sensorineural hearing loss
   c. facial nerve paralysis
   d. all of the above

3. A patient has a 40 dB hearing loss caused by otosclerosis in the left ear. Acoustic reflexes with contralateral stimulation would probably show
   a. absent right, absent left
   b. present right, present left
   c. present right, absent left
   d. absent right, present left

4. Flat tympanograms may be attributed to any of the following except
   a. otitis media
   b. impacted cerumen
   c. interrupted ossicular chain
   d. probe opening against canal wall

5. A retracted tympanic membrane should yield a tympanogram type
   a. A
   b. B
   c. C
   d. D

6. Of the following, the most likely tympanogram to occur in the presence of otosclerosis is
   a. A_S
   b. A_D
   c. B
   d. C

7. A measured increase in compliance of the tympanic membrane may result from
   a. interrupted ossicular chain
   b. middle-ear infection
   c. perforated tympanic membrane
   d. cerumenosis

8. An acoustic reflex at a sensation level below 55 dB suggests
   a. no pathology
   b. middle-ear pathology
   c. cochlear pathology
   d. auditory nerve pathology

9. The portion of the ear responsible for the stiffness component of impedance in the plane of the tympanic membrane is the
   a. external ear
   b. ossicular ligaments
   c. ossicular mass
   d. fluid load on the stapes

10. Theoretically, an interrupted ossicular chain shows the tympanogram type
   a. A
   b. A_S
   c. A_D
   d. C

11. A tympanogram with maximum compliance at −200 daPa suggests
   a. normally aerated middle ear
   b. negative pressure in the middle ear
   c. positive pressure in the middle ear
   d. fluid in the middle ear

12. According to the impedance formula, early otosclerosis should result in an audiometric configuration that is
   a. basically flat
   b. worse in the high frequencies
   c. worse in the mid-frequencies
   d. worse in the low frequencies

13. A tympanogram with no point of maximum compliance could result from
   a. fluid in the middle ear
   b. negative pressure in the middle ear
   c. a normally aerated middle ear
   d. positive pressure in the middle ear

14. In the use of an immittance meter with the probe in the right ear and the phone over the left ear, the contralateral acoustic reflex is designed to measure the
   a. Vth nerve left, reflex SL right
   b. recruitment right, decruitment left
   c. facial nerve left, reflex SL right
   d. facial nerve right, reflex SL left

15. Your patient has an intra-axial brain stem lesion on the right side but normal hearing for pure tones in both ears. Acoustic reflex results should be as follows:

    a. Contralateral: present left, absent right
       Ipsilateral: present left, present right

    b. Contralateral: present right, present left
       Ipsilateral: absent right, present left

    c. Contralateral: absent right, absent left
       Ipsilateral: present right, present left

    d. Contralateral: present right, present left
       Ipsilateral: absent right, absent left

16. Acoustic reflexes at 5 dB SL suggest

    a. retrocochlear lesion
    b. cochlear lesion
    c. conductive lesion
    d. nonorganic hearing loss

17. The tympanic membrane is maximally compliant when

    a. middle-ear pressure equals outer-ear pressure
    b. middle-ear pressure is less than outer-ear pressure
    c. middle-ear pressure is greater than outer-ear pressure
    d. all of the above

18. Reflex decay to half amplitude at 500 Hz within 10 seconds suggests

    a. normal hearing
    b. conductive lesion
    c. cochlear lesion
    d. retrocochlear lesion

19. During measurements of static compliance, a patient's C_1 reading is 5.0 cc. This suggests

    a. interrupted ossicular chain
    b. otosclerosis
    c. tympanic membrane perforation
    d. otitis media

20. The component of impedance unrelated to frequency is

    a. resistance
    b. mass
    c. stiffness
    d. pi

21. Present in the contralateral acoustic reflex pathway but absent in the ipsilateral acoustic reflex pathway are the
   a. cochlear nuclei
   b. crossover pathways
   c. auditory nerves
   d. superior olivary complexes

22. Auditory brain stem response audiometry views responses to sounds that occur
   a. almost immediately after the stimulus
   b. 350 msec after the stimulus
   c. visually
   d. never

23. One very important device for performing auditory evoked response audiometry is a(n)
   a. psychogalvanometer
   b. Wheatstone bridge
   c. averaging computer
   d. inductorium

24. During electrocochleography, the target electrode is not placed on the
   a. round window
   b. promontory
   c. external auditory canal
   d. mastoid process

25. During ABR the most reliable wave in normal hearing adults is number
   a. III
   b. IV
   c. V
   d. VI

26. Middle latency responses are those that occur ___ msec after the presentation of the signal
   a. 0–15
   b. 10–50
   c. 50–100
   d. 100–300

27. The usual stimulus for ABR is a
   a. click or tone burst
   b. pure tone
   c. narrowband noise
   d. broadband noise

28. During ABR the average electrical response is
    a. 1–5 millivolts
    b. 1–5 microvolts
    c. 1–5 volts
    d. none of the above

29. ECochG has an advantage over ABR in that
    a. bone conduction can be done without masking
    b. the test is less involved
    c. the test takes less time
    d. subjects need not be anesthetized

30. ABR results are an indication of
    a. neural integrity
    b. hearing loss in the 250 to 500 Hz range
    c. hearing loss in the 6000 to 8000 Hz range
    d. cortical function

31. The event-related potential is also called the
    a. ABR
    b. P300
    c. AMLR
    d. ECochG

32. Otoacoustic emissions occurring in the absence of external stimulation are called
    a. SOAE
    b. TEOAE
    c. EOAE
    d. DPOAE

33. Two primary tones are required when measuring
    a. SOAE
    b. TEOAE
    c. EOAE
    d. DPOAE

34. Otoacoustic emissions are usually absent in
    a. cochlear hearing loss
    b. conductive hearing loss
    c. VIIIth nerve hearing loss
    d. a and b

35. A patient with a moderate hearing loss and present evoked otoacoustic emissions probably has a(n)

    a. cochlear lesion

    b. conductive loss

    c. mixed loss

    d. VIIIth nerve loss

36. A patient with a mild-to-moderate sensorineural hearing loss with unexpectedly poor speech-recognition scores, absence of all auditory brain stem responses, and normal otoacoustic emissions, probably has

    a. auditory neuropathy

    b. cochlear hearing loss

    c. acoustic neuroma

    d. conductive hearing loss

VOCABULARY

acoustic impedance (Z)

acoustic reflex (AR)

acoustic reflex threshold (ART)

admittance

auditory brain stem response (ABR)

brain stem evoked response (BER)

cognitive response

compliance

distortion product otoacoustic
  emission (DPOAE)

electrocochleography (ECochG)

electrodermal audiometry (EDA)

equivalent volume

eustachian tube function test

facial nerve

immittance

intra-aural muscle reflex

late evoked response (LER)

middle ear (ME)

middle latency response (MLR)

ossicular chain

otoacoustic emission (OAE)

P300

physical volume test (PVT)

reactance

reflex decay

resistance

SPAR test

stapedius muscle

tensor tympani muscle

transient evoked otoacoustic emission
  (TEOAE)

tympanic membrane (TM)

tympanogram

tympanometry

ANSWERS

Matching	*Outline*	
1. e	**1.** B	**23.** E
2. o	**2.** D	**24.** C
3. i	**3.** H	**25.** V
4. s	**4.** K	**26.** AC
5. v	**5.** N	**27.** E
6. k	**6.** O	**28.** C
7. b	**7.** P	**29.** S
8. u	**8.** Q	**30.** AB
9. t	**9.** R	**31.** T
10. g	**10.** F	**32.** C
11. r	**11.** G	**33.** V
12. n	**12.** J	**34.** AD
13. q	**13.** M	
14. c	**14.** W	
15. d	**15.** X	
16. f	**16.** Y	
17. j	**17.** Z	
18. p	**18.** AA	
19. a	**19.** A	
20. h	**20.** I	
21. l	**21.** L	
22. m	**22.** U	

Activity

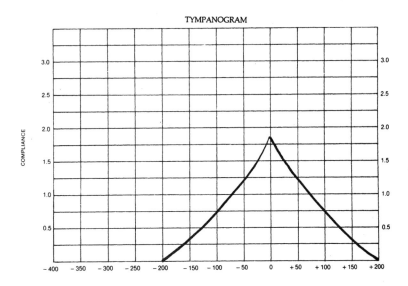

FIGURE 14.5 Type A

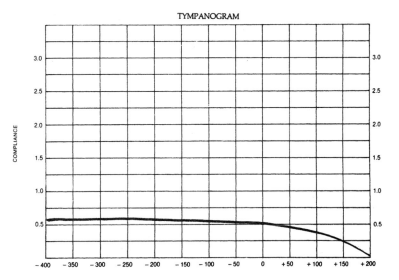

FIGURE 14.6 Type B

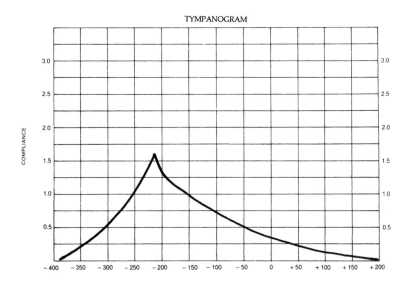

FIGURE 14.7   Type C

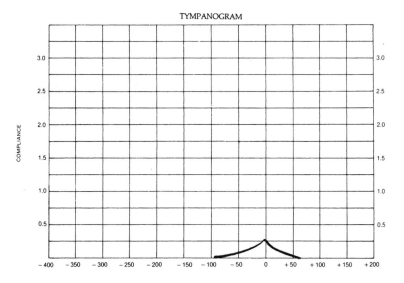

FIGURE 14.8   Type A$_s$

Multiple Choice

1. c		**19.** c
2. d		**20.** a
3. a		**21.** b
4. c		**22.** a
5. c		**23.** c
6. a		**24.** d
7. a		**25.** c
8. c		**26.** b
9. d		**27.** a
10. c		**28.** b
11. b		**29.** a
12. d		**30.** a
13. a		**31.** b
14. d		**32.** a
15. c		**33.** d
16. d		**34.** d
17. a		**35.** d
18. d		**36.** a

THE OUTER EAR

BACKGROUND

When laypersons think of the "ear," it is the outer ear that comes to mind. The outer ear is the most visible part of the auditory system and is made up primarily of a funnel-like appendage (the auricle, or pinna), a resonating tube (the external auditory canal), and a vibrating membrane (the tympanic membrane). The function of the auricle is to gather sound waves from the environment and allow them to propagate, via the external auditory canal, to the tympanic membrane. Anything that obstructs the passageway can cause a conductive hearing loss.

The outer ear is the conduit by which sounds from the environment are first introduced to the hearing mechanism. When portions of the outer ear are abnormal or diseased, hearing may or may not become impaired, depending on which structures are involved and the nature of their involvement. Some of the outer-ear structures found in humans are absent in such animals as birds and frogs, whose hearing sensitivity is nevertheless similar to that of humans. It is, of course, the outer ear of humans with which this unit is concerned.

Abnormalities of the external ear do not affect the sensorineural mechanism. However, alterations in the external auditory canal may cause a change in the osseotympanic mode of bone conduction, which may alter the bone-conduction curve slightly. Audiometric findings on speech recognition and site-of-lesion tests are the same as expected for persons with normal hearing. Measurements using an acoustic immittance meter are frequently impossible in external-ear anomalies, by virtue of the disorders themselves.

Disorders of the auricle surely affect the way people hear, but these differences are not demonstrated on usual auditory tests because the earphones ignore the auricle. For that reason people with missing or malformed pinnas are often thought to have no hearing problems at all when in fact their ability to hear certain high-frequency sounds, as well as their localization of sounds, may be impaired. Damaged or missing auricles may arise because of genetic factors, burns, frostbite, cancer, or trauma, and they can be quite disfiguring.

Disorders of the external auditory canal usually come about because of occlusion. Sometimes the canal is blocked by bone and/or cartilage caused by a congenital disorder called external auditory canal atresia. Blockage can also be brought about by swelling from disease or infection, obstruction by a foreign body (children are fond of putting precious items like crayons and pencil erasers into their ears), extreme narrowing of the canal, called stenosis, overaccumulations of earwax, and many other causes.

There is debate over whether the tympanic membrane should be considered a part of the outer ear or the middle ear. If the middle ear is thought of as a drum (the tympanum), then the tympanic membrane is the drumhead, or eardrum membrane. The tympanic membrane is often called the eardrum, when actually it is the entire middle ear that is the eardrum. This argument is relatively unrewarding, and it is like debating whether a door that separates two rooms is a part of one room or the other when it is actually part of both. So it is with the tympanic membrane.

The most common abnormality of the tympanic membrane that causes hearing loss is perforation. Perforations can be caused by pressure from infectious or noninfectious fluids in the middle ear or trauma. A common cause of perforation is overzealous use of cotton swabs in the external auditory canal. Sudden changes in air or water pressure can also traumatize the tympanic membrane. Tympanic membranes may become thickened by middle-ear disease or flaccid due to exposure to large pressure changes from activities like flying, skydiving, or SCUBA diving.

Whenever an audiologist sees a patient with an external-ear disorder, an otological consultation should be recommended. If hearing is impaired and no medical therapy is available, audiological treatment options should be investigated, depending on the extent of hearing loss and the needs of the patient. These may include the use of hearing aids or educational considerations for children. If the pinna is missing or deformed, there are often serious psychological considerations that should not be ignored.

OBJECTIVES

1. You should know and understand the terms in the matching exercise.

2. You should be able to fill in the outline, selecting items from the list provided.

3. You should be able to label parts of the outer ear and tympanic membrane in Figures 15.1, 15.2, and 15.3.

4. You should be able to answer the multiple-choice questions and understand the anatomy and physiology of the outer ear, as well as the causes of disorders that produce conductive hearing loss.

5. You should know and understand the terms in the vocabulary list and be able to describe or define each term.

MATCHING

Match the term from the column on the right with its definition.

Definition

1. ___ Earwax

2. ___ A special light designed for looking into the ear

3. ___ Absence of the pinna

4. ___ The same as pars flaccida

5. ___ Inflammation of the external ear

6. ___ The tense portion of the tympanic membrane, making up its largest area and consisting of three layers

7. ___ The appendage of the external ear consisting of cartilage

8. ___ Surgery to repair the tympanic membrane

9. ___ The point of the tympanic membrane that is approximately in the center

10. ___ Closure of a body orifice that is normally open

11. ___ The flabby portion of the tympanic membrane found near the top

12. ___ The membrane that vibrates to allow sound to enter the middle ear from the outer ear

13. ___ Ear pain

14. ___ The channel that conducts sound from the auricle to the tympanic membrane

15. ___ Failure of a portion of the anatomy to develop

Term

a. Agenesis

b. Anotia

c. Atresia

d. Auricle

e. Cerumen

f. External auditory canal

g. External otitis

h. Myringoplasty

i. Otalgia

j. Otoscope

k. Pars flaccida

l. Pars tensa

m. Shrapnell's membrane

n. Tympanic membrane

o. Umbo

OUTLINE

The Outer Ear

Anatomy

1. ___

2. ___

3. ___

4. ___

Disorders

5. ___

6. ___

7. ___

8. ___

9. ___

10. ___

Surgical Treatment

11. ___

12. ___

Select From

A. Atresia

B. Bony external ear canal

C. Cartilaginous external ear canal

D. Foreign bodies

E. Infections

F. Myringoplasty

G. Perforations

H. Pinna

I. Tympanic membrane

J. Tympanoplasty

K. Tumors

L. Wax impaction

ACTIVITIES

Label the parts of the pinna, outer ear, and tympanic membrane in Figures 15.1, 15.2, and 15.3. Select the terms from the lists provided.

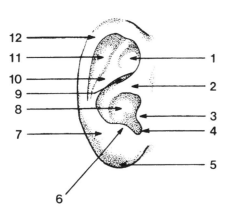

FIGURE 15.1 **The pinna (auricle)**

Label	Term
1. ___	**A.** Antihelix
2. ___	**B.** Antitragus
3. ___	**C.** Cavum concha
4. ___	**D.** Crus of helix
5. ___	**E.** Cymba concha
6. ___	**F.** Helix
7. ___	**G.** Intertragal notch
8. ___	**H.** Lobe
9. ___	**I.** Scaphoid fossa
10. ___	**J.** Tragus
11. ___	**K.** Triangular fossa
12. ___	

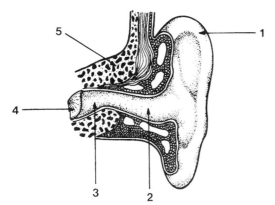

FIGURE 15.2 **The outer ear**

Label	Term
1. ___	**A.** Auricle (pinna)
2. ___	**B.** Bony external auditory canal
3. ___	**C.** Cartilaginous external auditory canal
4. ___	**D.** Mastoid air cells
5. ___	**E.** Tympanic membrane

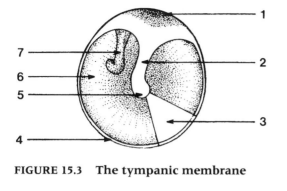

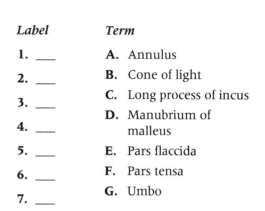

Label	Term
1. ___	**A.** Annulus
2. ___	**B.** Cone of light
3. ___	**C.** Long process of incus
4. ___	**D.** Manubrium of malleus
5. ___	**E.** Pars flaccida
6. ___	**F.** Pars tensa
7. ___	**G.** Umbo

FIGURE 15.3   The tympanic membrane

MULTIPLE CHOICE

1. Cerumen is produced in the
   a. entire external auditory canal
   b. cartilaginous external auditory canal
   c. osseous external auditory canal
   d. temporomandibular joint

2. Congenital absence of the external auditory canal is called
   a. microtia
   b. stenosis
   c. minutia
   d. atresia

3. The portion of the tympanic membrane in which the malleus is embedded is the
   a. umbo
   b. annulus
   c. cone of light
   d. pars tensa

4. A large central perforation of the tympanic membrane theoretically results in hearing that is
   a. normal
   b. slightly to moderately impaired
   c. severely impaired
   d. profoundly impaired

5. A term for a bacterial infection of the outer ear is
   a. otomycosis
   b. cerumen in the lumen
   c. otitis media
   d. external otitis

6. The portion of the tympanic membrane that does not contain the fibrocartilaginous layer is the
   a. umbo
   b. pars tensa
   c. pars flaccida
   d. annulus

7. In air-conduction audiometry, a loss of the pinna results in
   a. no measurable hearing loss
   b. mild sensorineural hearing loss
   c. mild conductive hearing loss
   d. mild mixed hearing loss

8. The point of maximum retraction of the tympanic membrane is the
   a. annulus
   b. concha
   c. umbo
   d. pars flaccida

9. The resonant frequency of the external auditory canal is
   a. 500–2000 Hz
   b. 3000–5000 Hz
   c. 8000–10,000 Hz
   d. 10,000–12,000 Hz

10. The innermost layer of the tympanic membrane (on the middle-ear side) is covered with
   a. epidermis
   b. fibrous material
   c. mucous membrane
   d. muscle

11. The cone of light of the tympanic membrane is
   a. superior-anterior
   b. superior-posterior
   c. inferior-anterior
   d. inferior-posterior

12. Narrowing of the external auditory canal is called

    a. atresia

    b. stenosis

    c. otitis

    d. otomycosis

VOCABULARY

agenesis	otalgia
anotia	otoscope
atresia	pars flaccida
auricle	pars tensa
cerumen	Shrapnell's membrane
external auditory canal	tympanic membrane
external otitis	umbo
myringoplasty	

ANSWERS

Matching	*Outline*	*Activities*
1. e	**1.** B	Pinna
2. j	**2.** C	**1.** K
3. b	**3.** H	**2.** D
4. m	**4.** I	**3.** J
5. g	**5.** A	**4.** G
6. l	**6.** D	**5.** H
7. d	**7.** E	**6.** B
8. h	**8.** G	**7.** F
9. o	**9.** K	**8.** C
10. c	**10.** L	**9.** E
11. k	**11.** F	**10.** A
12. n	**12.** J	**11.** I
13. i		**12.** F
14. f		
15. a		

Outer Ear

1. A
2. C
3. B
4. E
5. D

Tympanic Membrane

1. E
2. D
3. B
4. A
5. G
6. F
7. C

Multiple Choice

1. b
2. d
3. d
4. b
5. d
6. c
7. a
8. c
9. b
10. c
11. c
12. b

PHYSICS OF SOUND

BACKGROUND

The study of audiology must begin with a basic understanding of the physics of sound and some of the properties of its measurement and perception. Humans are accustomed to hearing sound as a wave disturbance propagated through air. Three properties are necessary to produce sound waves: a force (something to set the sound source into vibration as when a tuning fork is struck against a firm surface [see Unit 20]), a vibrating mass (such as the tines of the tuning fork), and an elastic medium (air being the primary medium conveying sounds that the human ear hears). Many factors may affect sound waves during their creation and propagation, and most are specified physically in terms of the frequency and intensity of vibrations. Human reactions to sound, like those of other animals, are psychological and reflect such subjective experiences as pitch, loudness, sound quality, and the ability to tell the direction of a sound source.

Whenever air molecules are disturbed by a body that is set into vibration, they move from the point of disturbance, striking and bouncing off adjacent molecules. Because of their elasticity, the original molecules bounce back after having forced their neighbors from their previous positions. When the molecules are pushed close together, they are said to be condensed or compressed. When a space exists between areas of compression, this area is said to be rarefied. The succession of molecules being shoved together and then pulled apart sets up the motion called waves. Sound waves, therefore, are made up of successive compressions and rarefactions.

Sound may be defined in terms of either psychological or physical phenomena. In the psychological sense a sound is an auditory experience—the act of hearing something. In the physical sense, sound is a series of disturbances of molecules within, and propagated through, an elastic medium such as air. Air molecules are the mass undergoing to-and-fro motion (vibration), and air itself has an elastic nature so that the molecules, in their vibratory motion, seem to be connected by springs moving away from the sound's source to strike adjacent molecules and then returning to their original positions. It is only when a sound pressure wave reaches the ear that hearing takes place.

Sound waves are produced by molecular vibration because of the pressure conditions that are created when molecules are compressed or rarefied. As molecules undergo oscillation, successive compressions, followed by rarefactions, are passed along the line of particles at a speed that is determined by the medium. The elasticity, or springiness, of any medium is increased as the distance between the molecules is decreased. The denser the medium, the faster adjacent molecules can be "bumped" and caused to move. Therefore, sound travels faster in a liquid than it does in a gas and faster in a solid than it does in a liquid. Sound may travel through any elastic medium, although our immediate concern is the propagation of sound in air.

Every cubic inch of the air that surrounds us is filled with billions and billions of tiny molecules. These particles move about randomly, constantly bouncing off one another, a phenomenon known as Brownian motion. The rate at which this random movement occurs is determined by the elasticity of the object and the heat in the environment.

Waves behaving with simple periodic oscillation are often called sine waves. These waves may be described, in part, in terms of how often they move from maximum rarefaction to maximum compression and then return to their point of origin; this is called the frequency of the wave. The measurement unit for frequency is cycles per second (cps) or hertz (Hz), named for the famed German physicist Heinrich Hertz. Frequency is interpreted psychologically as pitch.

The intensity of a wave is the force that moves it to its maximum amplitude. The measurement unit for intensity is the decibel (dB), which is one tenth of a Bel, named for Alexander Graham Bell, renowned Scottish teacher of deaf children and inventor of the telephone. The decibel is a ratio between two sound pressures or two sound powers.

Waves of different frequencies may combine to form interactions called complex waves. Different complex waveforms produce the quality or timbre of a sound. Speech is an example of a complex wave. The complexities of the production of human speech and its propagation through air pales in comparison to the complexities underlying the reception and consequent perception of speech by the brain (e.g., see Units 8 and 11).

OBJECTIVES

1. You should know and understand the terms in the matching exercise.

2. You should be able to fill in the outline, selecting items from the list provided.

3. You should be able to label the different parts of Figure 16.1 relating to sound waves.

4. You should be able to do the matching exercise on sound measurement units.

5. You should be able to answer the multiple-choice questions on the physics of sound.

6. You should know and understand the terms in the vocabulary list and be able to describe or define each term.

MATCHING 1

Match the term from the column on the right with its definition.

Definition

1. ___ The ability of a mass to return to its natural shape

2. ___ The exponent that tells the power to which a number is raised

3. ___ A unit of power

4. ___ A whole-number multiple of the fundamental of a complex wave

5. ___ The extent of the vibratory movement of a mass to the point furthest from its position of rest

6. ___ The portion of a sound wave where the molecules become less dense

7. ___ The amount of sound energy per unit of area

8. ___ The duration of one cycle of vibration

9. ___ A unit of expressing ratios in base 10 logarithms

10. ___ The waveform of a pure tone showing simple harmonic motion

11. ___ The difference between tones separated by a frequency ratio of 2:1

12. ___ The speed of a sound wave in a given direction

13. ___ A unit of pitch measurement

14. ___ The to-and-fro movements of a mass

15. ___ The distance between the same points on two successive cycles of a tone

16. ___ Reduction in amplitude to zero because of interaction of two tones 180 degrees out of phase

17. ___ The number of complete oscillations of a vibrating body per unit of time

18. ___ A series of moving impulses set up by a vibration

Term

a.   Amplitude

b.   Aperiodic wave

c.   Beats

d.   Bel

e.   Brownian motion

f.   Cancellation

g.   Component

h.   Compression

i.   Cosine wave

j.   Damping

k.   Difference tone

l.   Dyne

m.   Elasticity

n.   Exponent

o.   Force

p.   Frequency

q.   Fundamental frequency

r.   Harmonic

s.   Intensity

t.   Logarithm

u.   Mel

v.   Microbar

w.   Newton

x.   Octave

y.   Oscillation

z.   Overtone

aa. Pascal

ab. Period

ac. Periodic wave

19. ___ Progressive lessening in the amplitude of a vibrating body

20. ___ The impetus required to increase the velocity of a vibrating body

21. ___ Periodic variations of the amplitude of a tone caused by a second tone of slightly different frequency

22. ___ A unit of pressure equal to 1 Newton per meter square

23. ___ A logarithm

24. ___ A unit of force just sufficient to accelerate a mass of 1 gram at 1 cm per second squared

25. ___ A pressure equal to one-millionth of standard atmospheric pressure

26. ___ The lowest frequency of vibration in a complex wave

27. ___ The frequency of a tone produced by two tones of slightly different frequency

28. ___ A waveform that does not repeat itself over time

29. ___ The relationship in time between two or more waves

30. ___ A force equal to 100,000 dynes

31. ___ The portion of a sound wave where molecules become more dense

32. ___ A pure tone constituent of a complex wave

33. ___ A unit of loudness measurement

34. ___ A waveform that repeats itself over time

35. ___ The constant colliding movement of molecules in a medium

36. ___ The unit of loudness level

37. ___ The ability of a mass to vibrate at a particular frequency with minimum external force

38. ___ A sound wave representing simple harmonic motion that begins at 90 or 270 degrees

39. ___ Like a harmonic but numbered differently

ad. Phase

ae. Phon

af. Rarefaction

ag. Resonance

ah. Sinusoid

ai. Sone

aj. Velocity

ak. Watt

al. Waves

am. Wavelength

OUTLINE

Physics of Sound	*Select From*
Waves	**A.** Complex
1. ___	**B.** Cycles per second
2. ___	**C.** Decibel
3. ___	**D.** Forced vibration
4. ___	**E.** Fourier analysis
Vibrations	**F.** Free vibration
5. ___	**G.** Hearing level
6. ___	**H.** Hertz
Frequency	**I.** Length effects
7. ___	**J.** Longitudinal
8. ___	**K.** Loudness
9. ___	**L.** Mass effects
10. ___	**M.** Pitch
Intensity	**N.** Power
11. ___	**O.** Pressure
12. ___	**P.** Quality
13. ___	**Q.** Sensation level
14. ___	**R.** Sine
Decibels	**S.** Sound-pressure level
15. ___	**T.** Transverse
16. ___	**U.** Work
17. ___	
Spectrum	
18. ___	
Psychological Acoustics	
19. ___	
20. ___	
21. ___	

ACTIVITY

Five parts of the sine wave shown in Figure 16.1 are labeled. Each part may be referred to in two ways. Label each part appropriately.

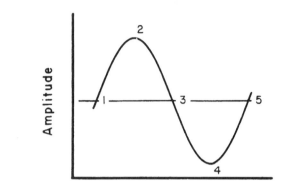

FIGURE 16.1   Sine wave

                                  Time/Degrees

Label		*Term*
1. ____ ____		**A.** Maximum amplitude
2. ____ ____		**B.** 90 degrees
3. ____ ____		**C.** 180 degrees
4. ____ ____		**D.** 360 degrees
5. ____ ____		**E.** 270 degrees
		F. Zero amplitude
		G. 0 degrees

MATCHING 2

Match the measurement unit to each measurement below.

Measurement	*Unit*
Acceleration	**a.** Centimeter (cm)
1. ___	**b.** Centimeter per second (cm/s)
2. ___	**c.** Centimeter per second squared (cm/s^2)
Area	**d.** Centimeter squared (cm^2)
3. ___	**e.** Dyne (dyn)
4. ___	**f.** Dyne per centimeter squared (dyn/cm^2)
Force	**g.** Erg (e)
5. ___	**h.** Ergs per second (e/s)
6. ___	**i.** Gram (g)
Intensity	**j.** Joule (J)
7. ___	**k.** Joules per second (J/s)
8. ___	**l.** Kilogram (kg)
Length	**m.** Meter (m)
9. ___	**n.** Meters per second (m/s)
10. ___	**o.** Meters per second squared (m/s^2)
Mass	**p.** Meter squared (m^2)
11. ___	**q.** Newton (N)
12. ___	**r.** Newton per meter squared (N/m^2)
Power	**s.** Pascal (Pa)
13. ___	**t.** Watt (W)
14. ___	**u.** Watt per centimeter squared (W/cm^2)
15. ___	**v.** Watt per meter squared (W/m^2)
Pressure	
16. ___	
17. ___	
18. ___	
Velocity	
19. ___	
20. ___	
Work	
21. ___	
22. ___	

MULTIPLE CHOICE

1. Sound intensity
   a. decreases linearly as a function of distance from the source
   b. decreases inversely as a function of the square of the distance from the source
   c. is unaffected by the distance from the source
   d. is the same in fluid as in gas

2. Wavelength is
   a. sound velocity divided by frequency
   b. sound frequency divided by velocity
   c. frequency divided by a constant
   d. determined by intensity

3. If the fifth harmonic of a sound is 500 Hz, the fundamental frequency is
   a. indeterminable from the above information
   b. determined by wavelength
   c. 250 Hz
   d. 100 Hz

4. The period of a 100 Hz tone is
   a. 1/1000 sec
   b. 1/100 sec
   c. 1/10 sec
   d. 1 sec

5. Acceleration is
   a. the same as velocity
   b. the same as speed
   c. velocity divided by time
   d. 0 to 60 mph in 9 sec

6. When the expression sound-pressure level (SPL) is used, this means that the reference is
   a. 10^{-16} watt/cm²
   b. 0.002 dyn/cm²
   c. 20 Pascals
   d. 20 micropascals

7. When the expression intensity level (IL) is used, this means that the reference is not
   a. 10^{-16} watt/cm²
   b. 10^{-12} watt/m²

    c. in decibels

    d. 0.0002 dyn/cm^2

8. The unit of measurement for pitch is the

    a. sone

    b. phon

    c. hertz

    d. mel

9. The SPL of a sound with a pressure output of 200 micropascals is

    a. 10 dB

    b. 20 dB

    c. 30 dB

    d. 40 dB

10. The IL of a sound is 50 dB. Its intensity output is

    a. 10^{-7} watt/m^2

    b. 100 dB

    c. 20 micropascals

    d. 0.0002 dyn/cm^2

11. The velocity of sound in air is said to be

    a. 20 mph

    b. 1,130 ft/sec

    c. 5,286 ft/sec

    d. 14.7 mph

12. Masking may take place when

    a. the masker precedes the signal

    b. the signal precedes the masker

    c. the masker and signal coexist in time

    d. all of the above

13. At its resonant frequency, a mass vibrates

    a. with the least amount of applied energy

    b. with the greatest amount of applied energy

    c. at its least possible amplitude

    d. as a free vibration

14. The condition in which air molecules are packed most tightly together is called the

    a. resonant frequency

    b. rarefaction

    c. sine wave

    d. compression

15. The quality of a sound is also called its
   a. phase
   b. pure tone
   c. timbre
   d. resonance

16. In the propagation of sound, as air molecules are moved further from each other, they are said to be
   a. condensed
   b. compressed
   c. inert
   d. rarefied

17. The log of 1 is
   a. 0
   b. 1
   c. 2
   d. 3

18. Sounds we hear may be the result of
   a. incident waves
   b. reflected waves
   c. composite waves
   d. all of the above

19. The velocity of sound is
   a. unaffected by the medium
   b. greater in denser media
   c. greater in less dense media
   d. none of the above

20. The joule is a unit of
   a. work
   b. power
   c. intensity
   d. frequency

21. The unit of measurement in equal loudness contours is
   a. mel
   b. sone
   c. decibel
   d. phon

VOCABULARY

amplitude	loudness
aperiodic wave	mel
beats	microbar
Bel	Newton
Brownian motion	octave
cancellation	oscillation
complex wave	overtone
component	Pascal
compression	period
cosine wave	periodic wave
cycle	phase
cycles per second (CPS)	phon
damping	pitch
decibel	power
difference tone	pressure
dyne	quality
elasticity	rarefaction
exponent	resonance
force	sinusoid
forced vibration	sone
free vibration	sound-pressure level (SPL)
frequency	velocity
fundamental frequency	vibration
harmonic	watt
hertz (Hz)	wave
intensity	wavelength
logarithm	work

ANSWERS

Matching 1		*Outline*	*Activity*
1. m	**21.** c	**1.** A	**1.** F
2. t	**22.** aa	**2.** J	G
3. ak	**23.** n	**3.** R	**2.** A
4. r	**24.** l	**4.** T	B
5. a	**25.** v	**5.** D	**3.** C
6. af	**26.** q	**6.** F	F
7. s	**27.** k	**7.** B	**4.** A
8. ab	**28.** b	**8.** H	E
9. d	**29.** ad	**9.** I	**5.** D
10. ah	**30.** w	**10.** L	F
11. x	**31.** h	**11.** C	
12. aj	**32.** g	**12.** N	
13. u	**33.** ai	**13.** O	
14. y	**34.** ac	**14.** U	
15. am	**35.** e	**15.** G	
16. f	**36.** ae	**16.** Q	
17. p	**37.** ag	**17.** S	
18. al	**38.** i	**18.** E	
19. j	**39.** z	**19.** K	
20. o		**20.** M	
		21. P	

Matching 2	*Multiple Choice*
1. c	**1.** b
2. o	**2.** a
3. d	**3.** d
4. p	**4.** b
5. e	**5.** c
6. q	**6.** d
7. u	**7.** d
8. v	**8.** d
9. a	**9.** b
10. m	**10.** a
11. i	**11.** b
12. l	**12.** d
13. h	**13.** a
14. k	**14.** d
15. t	**15.** c
16. f	**16.** d
17. r	**17.** a
18. s	**18.** d
19. b	**19.** b
20. n	**20.** a
21. g	**21.** d
22. j	

PROFESSIONAL CONSIDERATIONS

BACKGROUND

Prior to World War II, hearing-care services were provided by physicians and commercial hearing-aid dealers. It was the influx of service personnel reentering civilian life during World War II that created the impetus for the development of audiometric techniques and rehabilitative procedures within military-based clinics and later the expansion of these services within the private sector. Over the next several decades audiology developed rapidly as a profession distinct from medicine in the United States, with most audiologists around the globe looking to U.S. audiologists for the model of autonomous practice that they wish to emulate. In the United States, educational preparation for audiologists has evolved as technology has expanded so that today's students graduate with a professional doctorate, the Au.D. The goal is to prepare graduates who are ready to tackle the responsibilities of a growing scope of practice, which includes the identification of hearing loss, the differential diagnosis of hearing impairment, and the nonmedical treatment of hearing and balance disorders.

A license to practice audiology or professional registration within a state constitutes the legal requirement to practice the profession of audiology in each of the fifty states of the union. Licensure and registration are important forms of consumer protection, and the loss or revocation of this documentation prohibits an individual from practicing audiology. In contrast to state licensure and registration, certification is not a legal requirement for the practice of audiology. Many audiologists chose to become certified either by the American Speech-Language-Hearing Association (a requirement for membership in this association) or by the American Board of Audiology, an independent certifying board. Either certification is an attestation that one holds him- or herself to a higher standard than may be set forth in the legal documents of licensure or registration.

It is generally accepted that there are more than 28 million people in the United States with sufficient hearing loss to affect their lives adversely with a prevalence that increases markedly with age. Even so, the prevalence of hearing loss in children is almost staggering if we consider those children whose speech and language development and academic performances may be impacted by even mild, transient ear infections so common among children. In addition to the personal effects of hearing loss on the individual—which may include reductions in educational performance, social isolation, frustration, and depression—the financial burden of hearing loss placed upon the individual, and society at large, is remarkable.

The blending of the science of audiology with the art of patient treatment makes audiology a highly rewarding profession that is practiced within a variety of settings, including medical facilities, schools, and private practices. Often an audiologist's chosen area of concentration dictates what professional societies he or she affiliates with. In addition to the parent associations of the American Academy of Audiology and the American Speech-Language-Hearing Association, audiologists may choose to be members of the American Auditory Society, the Academy of Dispensing Audiologists, the Academy of Rehabilitative Audiology, the Educational Audiology Association, or one or more of the primarily consumer-oriented associations such as Self Help for Hard of Hearing People, Inc. (SHHH) and the Alexander Graham Bell Association for the Deaf.

OBJECTIVES

1. You should know and understand the terms in the matching exercise.

2. You should be able to fill in the outline, selecting items from the list provided.

3. You should be able to answer the multiple choice questions and recognize the varying responsibilities of audiologists within different specialty areas.

4. You should know and understand the terms in the vocabulary list and be able to describe or define each term.

MATCHING

Match the term from the column on the right with its definition.

Definition

1. ___ The branch of medicine devoted to the study, diagnosis, and treatment of diseases of the ear and related structures

2. ___ The treatment of those with hearing loss that has begun after birth, usually after speech and language development, to improve overall communication ability

3. ___ An organization that adopted the new discipline of audiology in 1947, providing audiology with its first professional home

4. ___ An organization founded in 1988, of, by, and for audiologists

5. ___ The number of existing cases of a disease or disorder in a given population at a given time

Term

a. AAA

b. ASHA

c. Aural rehabilitation

d. Otology

e. Prevalence

OUTLINE

The Profession

Audiology Specialties

1. ___

2. ___

3. ___

4. ___

5. ___

Professional Associations

6. ___

7. ___

8. ___

9. ___

10. ___

11. ___

Select From

A. American Academy of Audiology

B. American Auditory Society

C. Academy of Dispensing Audiologists

D. Academy of Rehabilitative Audiology

E. American Speech-Language-Hearing Association

F. Educational

G. Educational Audiology Association

H. Hearing aid dispensing/ Rehabilitation

I. Industrial

J. Medical

K. Pediatric

MULTIPLE CHOICE

1. At its origin, audiology pooled its knowledge base from
   a. otology
   b. speech pathology
   c. psychology
   d. all of the above

2. The prevalence of hearing loss
   a. decreases over time
   b. increases with age
   c. is unknown
   d. is at an all-time low thanks to modern medical practice

3. The impact of hearing loss
   a. is greater for more severe hearing loss
   b. can affect social maturation
   c. may create an economic burden in excess of one million dollars across an individual's lifetime
   d. all of the above

4. The organization that provided the first "home" for the profession of audiology was
   a. AAS (American Auditory Society)
   b. ARA (Academy of Rehabilitative Audiology)
   c. ASHA (American Speech-Language-Hearing Association)
   d. AAA (American Academy of Audiology)

5. The word *audiology*
   a. means the study of hearing
   b. combines the Latin root, *audire*, with the Greek suffix, *logos*
   c. is often reported to have been coined by the "Father of Audiology," Dr. Raymond Carhart
   d. all of the above

VOCABULARY

Academy of Rehabilitative Audiology (ARA)

Academy of Dispensing Audiologists (ADA)

American Academy of Audiology (AAA)

American Auditory Society (AAS)

American Speech-Language-Hearing Association (ASHA)

audiology

auditory rehabilitation

educational audiology

Educational Audiology Association

hearing aid dispensing

industrial audiology

medical audiology

otolaryngology

otology

pediatric audiology

prevalence

ANSWERS

Matching	*Outline*	*Multiple Choice*
1. d	**1.** F	**1.** d
2. c	**2.** H	**2.** b
3. b	**3.** I	**3.** d
4. a	**4.** J	**4.** c
5. e	**5.** K	**5.** d
	6. A	
	7. B	
	8. C	
	9. D	
	10. E	
	11. G	

PURE-TONE AUDIOMETRY

BACKGROUND

The audiogram is a graph that depicts a patient's thresholds of audibility for a se-ries of pure tones. The graph is arranged so that intensity (in dB HL) is shown on the ordinate. The lower on the graph, the greater the intensity, with 0 dB HL near the top and 110 dB HL near the bottom. Frequency is shown on the abscissa. The further to the right, the higher the frequency, with 125 Hz usually on the left and 8000 Hz on the right. A patient's auditory thresholds are measured for each ear by air conduction (AC) with the use of earphones. Thresholds are also measured by bone conduction (BC), using a special oscillator.

Thresholds are displayed on the audiogram using symbols, as shown on a key on the audiogram form. For AC and forehead BC the symbol is placed on the vertical line indicating the frequency tested where it intersects the horizontal line, showing the intensity required to reach threshold. If mastoid BC testing is done (with or without masking), or forehead BC is done with masking, the symbol is placed to the left of the vertical line for the right ear's response and to the right of the vertical line for the left ear's response as if the audiogram were the patient's face looking up. Red is used for the right ear and blue for the left ear. The AC threshold for each frequency reveals the total amount of hearing loss while the BC threshold reveals the amount of hearing loss (if any) that is sensorineural. The amount by which hearing by AC is poorer than hearing by BC, the air-bone gap (ABG), reveals the conductive component. AC symbols should be connected with a solid line and BC symbols may either not be connected or may be connected with a dashed line. Audiograms may reveal normal hearing, conductive hearing loss, sensorineural hearing loss, or mixed hearing loss.

After thresholds are determined on a patient, they are compared to estab-lished norms (usually −10 to 15 dB HL) at all frequencies tested. Audiometers are equipped to test hearing sensitivity by air conduction and bone conduction. A switch allows for selection of pure tones. The testable frequencies for air conduc-tion usually include 125, 250, 500, 750, 1000, 1500, 2000, 3000, 4000, 6000, and

8000 Hz. The range of intensities begins at −10 dB HL and goes to 110 dB HL at frequencies between 500 and 6000 Hz, with slightly lower maximum values at 125, 250, and 8000 Hz. A matched pair of earphones or insert receiver housings (color coded red for the right phone and blue for the left phone) is provided and an output switch directs the tone to either earphone.

There is no resolution to the debate about how degrees of hearing loss should be classified. An approach based on empirical evidence suggests that a hearing threshold higher (greater) than 15 dB HL can and should be considered to be handicapping. We believe 16 to 25 dB to be a slight loss, 26 to 40 dB a mild loss, 41 to 55 dB a moderate loss, 56 to 70 dB a moderately severe loss, 71 to 90 dB severe, and greater than 90 dB profound.

Usually only the range from 250 through 4000 Hz may be tested by bone conduction. The maximum testable hearing level for bone conduction is considerably lower than for air conduction, not exceeding 50 dB at 250 Hz and 70 or 80 dB at 500 Hz and above. Maximum outputs for bone conduction are lower than for air conduction for several reasons. The power required to drive a bone-conduction oscillator is greater than for an air-conduction earphone. In addition, when the bone-conduction oscillator is driven at high intensities, harmonic distortion takes place, especially in the low frequencies. Finally, high-intensity sounds delivered by a bone-conduction oscillator may result in the patient feeling, rather than hearing the stimulus.

In addition to air- and bone-conduction capability, a masking control is usually provided that allows for introduction of a noise to the nontest ear when needed during audiometry. For some audiometers, the masking noise is not of a specific spectrum and is not well calibrated for practical clinical purposes. Persons who rely solely on portable air- and bone-conduction audiometers are often unsophisticated about the need for and proper use of masking. Most pure-tone audiometers, however, contain excellent masking-noise generators and can be used for a variety of pure-tone audiometric procedures (see Unit 9).

A maximum ambient sound-pressure level is allowable for accurate air-conduction and bone-conduction testing. Rooms in which such standards can be met are not always utilized. This is true in the case of hearing-test sites in industry or in the public schools. Regardless of the practical limitations imposed by a given situation, the person responsible for audiometric results must realize that background noise may affect audiometric results by elevating auditory thresholds or causing unnecessary screening failures. There are three major ways in which ambient room noise may be attenuated: by using specially designed earphone enclosures, by testing through receivers that insert into the ear, and by using sound-treated chambers.

The audiometer earphone and cushion combinations that accompany most audiometers do not provide sufficient attenuation of most background noises to allow the determination of threshold down to 0 dB HL for people with normal hearing. Several devices are available that allow the supra-aural audiometer ear-phone and cushion to be mounted within a larger cup, which assists in the atten-uation of background noise. Most use a fluid-filled cushion to achieve a tight seal against the head. Such enclosures may be effective, but differences exist in the ef-ficiency of different devices.

Testing hearing with receivers that insert directly into the ear has a number of advantages audiometrically. When the foam tips are placed into the ears, atten-uation of background noise is increased compared to the supra-aural earphone-cushion arrangement. If the foam is inserted deep into the ear, even more attenuation is obtained. It is desirable to have patients open and close their mouths three or four times to ensure proper seating of the cushion. Insert earphones can be used for testing children as well as adults. Problems with room-noise masking remain unsolved for bone-conduction testing, even if insert earphones are used for air conduction, since ears must be uncovered during bone-conduction testing.

Despite the development of remarkable procedures for the measurement of human hearing, pure-tone audiometry remains the gold standard. Speech-language pathologists should see to it that all their patients, regardless of the rea-son for treatment, have audiometric tests carried out.

OBJECTIVES

1. You should know and understand the terms in the matching exercise.

2. You should be able to fill in the outline, selecting items from the list provided.

3. You should memorize the symbols used in plotting an audiogram, including those for right and left ear air conduction and bone conduction. You should also know the symbols to use when masking is used in the opposite ear.

4. You should be able to draw an audiogram based on a patient's thresholds for air conduction and bone conduction.

5. You should be able to interpret audiograms in terms of the type and degree of hearing loss.

6. You should be able to answer the multiple-choice questions and understand the purpose and use of the audiogram.

7. You should know and understand the terms in the vocabulary list and be able to describe or define each term.

MATCHING

Match the term from the column on the right with its definition.

Definition

1. ___ The horizontal line on an audiogram or other graph

2. ___ A device for determining the thresholds of hearing

3. ___ The testing of hearing by specially programmed computer-driven audiometers

4. ___ Measurement made of hearing sensitivity by using earphones

5. ___ Failure of a patient to respond to a stimulus that has been heard

6. ___ The average of a patient's thresholds obtained at 500, 1000, and 2000 Hz

7. ___ The level at which a stimulus is barely perceptible 50 percent of the time

8. ___ Measurement made that tests hearing sensitivity exclusive of the outer and middle ears

9. ___ The amount of sound energy (in decibels) by which the air-conduction threshold exceeds the bone-conduction threshold

10. ___ A graph representing hearing sensitivity (in decibels) as a function of frequency

11. ___ A response during testing when no stimulus has been presented or was presented below the hearing threshold of the subject

12. ___ Testing hearing by having subjects track their own thresholds

13. ___ The vertical line on an audiogram or other graph

Term

a. Abscissa

b. Air-bone gap

c. Air conduction

d. Audiogram

e. Audiometer

f. Békésy audiometry

g. Bone conduction

h. Computerized audiometry

i. Ordinate

j. False negative

k. False positive

l. Pure-tone average

m. Threshold

OUTLINE

Audiogram Interpretation	*Select From*
The Graph	**A.** AC threshold
Abscissa	**B.** Blue
1. ____	**C.** BC threshold
Ordinate	**D.** Equal amount of loss for AC and BC
2. ____	**E.** 15 dB threshold or lower for AC
3. ____	**F.** Frequency
4. ____	**G.** Greater hearing loss by AC, with lesser hearing loss by BC
Code Color	**H.** Hearing loss by AC, normal hearing by BC
Right Ear	**I.** Intensity in dB HL
5. ____	**J.** Red
Left Ear	**K.** ○ (red)
6. ____	**L.** Δ (red)
Audiogram Types	**M.** < (red)
Normal Hearing	**N.** [(red)
7. ____	**O.** × (blue)
Audiogram Interpretation	**P.** □ (blue)
Conductive Hearing Loss	**Q.** > (blue)
8. ____	**R.**] (blue)
Sensorineural Hearing Loss	**S.** ∨ (black)
9. ____	**T.** ⌐ (red)
Mixed Hearing Loss	**U.** ⌐ (blue)
10. ____	

Symbols

Right Ear AC

   11. _____ (unmasked)

   12. _____ (masked)

Right Ear Mastoid BC

   13. _____ (unmasked)

   14. _____ (masked)

Left Ear AC

   15. _____ (unmasked)

   16. _____ (masked)

Left Ear Mastoid BC

   17. _____ (unmasked)

   18. _____ (masked)

Forehead BC

   19. _____ (unmasked)

   20. _____ Right (left ear marked)

   21. _____ Left (right ear masked)

ACTIVITY

Given the four sets of audiometric data below, draw the audiograms that follow (Figures 18.1 to 18.4), illustrating four basic conditions. Use the symbol indicating masking when an asterisk (*) is shown. Compare your graphs to the properly drawn audiograms (Figures 18.5 to 18.8) at the end of this unit.

TABLE 18.1   Audiometric Data

	RIGHT EAR						LEFT EAR					
	250	*500*	*1000*	*2000*	*4000*	*8000*	*250*	*500*	*1000*	*2000*	*4000*	*8000*
AC	40	40	35	40	45	40	35	45	40	40	50	45
BC	−5*	0*	5*	10*	0*	–	0*	0*	5*	5*	0*	–
AC	65	70	70	75	65	75	70	65	70	70	70	75
BC	25*	30*	35*	40*	50*	–	25*	30*	40*	50*	55*	–
AC	0	5	0	5	5	10	5	5	0	−5	0	5
BC	0	0	0	5	5	–	0	5	0	0	0	–
AC	25	30	35	35	50	60	30	40	45	50	60	55
BC	25	35	40	40	55	–	25	35	40	45	55	–

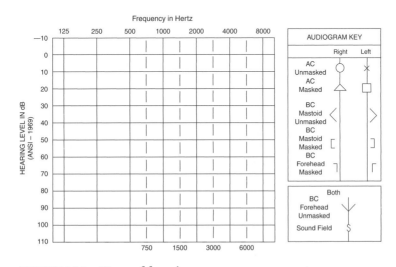

FIGURE 18.1   Normal hearing

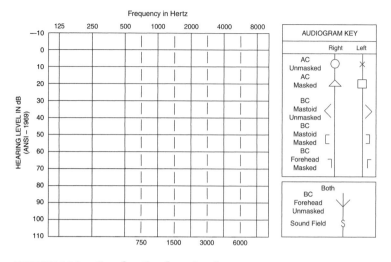

FIGURE 18.2   Conductive hearing loss

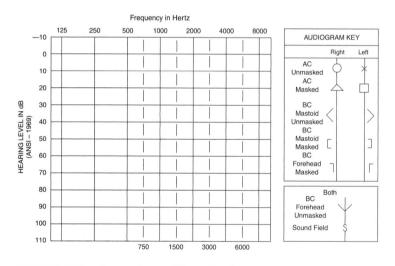

FIGURE 18.3   Sensorineural hearing loss

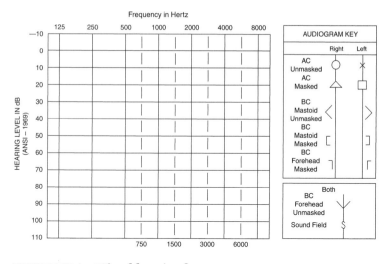

FIGURE 18.4 Mixed hearing loss

MULTIPLE CHOICE

1. The audiogram showing a conductive type of hearing loss will indicate
   a. impaired bone conduction, normal air conduction
   b. impaired air conduction, normal bone conduction
   c. impaired bone conduction, impaired air conduction
   d. normal bone conduction, normal air conduction

2. The audiogram showing a mixed type of hearing loss will indicate
   a. impaired bone conduction and an air-bone gap
   b. impaired air conduction and no air-bone gap
   c. impaired bone conduction and no air-bone gap
   d. normal bone conduction and an air-bone gap

3. The frequency range for bone conduction on most audiometers is
   a. 125–6000 Hz
   b. 250–8000 Hz
   c. 250–4000 Hz
   d. 125–8000 Hz

4. The maximum testable hearing level for bone conduction on an audiometer is usually
   a. the same as for air conduction
   b. greater than for air conduction
   c. less than for air conduction
   d. both a and c

5. The audiogram showing a sensorineural hearing loss will indicate
   a. impaired bone conduction and an air-bone gap
   b. impaired air conduction and no air-bone gap
   c. impaired bone conduction and normal air conduction
   d. normal bone conduction and an air-bone gap

6. The frequency range for air conduction on most audiometers is
   a. 125–6000 Hz
   b. 250–8000 Hz
   c. 250–4000 Hz
   d. 125–8000 Hz

7. For Figure 18.4 at 500 Hz, the conductive portion of the hearing loss in the right ear is ___ dB
   a. 70
   b. 30
   c. 40
   d. 35

8. For Figure 18.3 at 2000 Hz, the conductive portion of the hearing loss in the right ear is ___ dB
   a. 45
   b. 0
   c. −5
   d. 5

9. For Figure 18.1 at 2000 Hz in the left ear, BC is 5 dB poorer than AC. This suggests
   a. normal variability and may be ignored
   b. a slight conductive hearing loss
   c. a slight sensorineural hearing loss
   d. a slight mixed hearing loss

10. For Figure 18.2 at 4000 Hz in the left ear, the loss is
    a. completely conductive
    b. completely sensorineural

    c. partially mixed

    d. indeterminable

11. In determining the traditional pure-tone average, the audiometric frequencies used are

    a. 250, 500, 1000 Hz

    b. 1000, 2000, 3000 Hz

    c. 500, 1000, 2000 Hz

    d. 250, 1000, 4000 Hz

12. An apparent sensorineural hearing loss with an air-bone gap only at 3000 and 4000 Hz is probably due to

    a. the occlusion effect

    b. cross hearing by air conduction

    c. acoustic radiations from the bone-conduction vibrator

    d. acoustic radiations from the air-conduction receiver

13. If an audiogram is properly constructed, the distance across of one octave should be the same as the distance down of

    a. 5 dB

    b. 10 dB

    c. 15 dB

    d. 20 dB

14. Tactile responses to pure tones may be seen when stimuli are

    a. bone conduction only

    b. air conduction only

    c. bone conduction and air conduction

    d. sound field

VOCABULARY

abscissa	intensity
air-bone gap (ABG)	mixed hearing loss
air conduction (AC)	normal hearing
audiogram	ordinate
bone conduction (BC)	pure tone
conductive hearing loss	sensorineural hearing loss
frequency	threshold of audibility
hearing level (HL)	

ANSWERS

Matching		*Outline*	
1.	a	**1.**	F
2.	e	**2.**	A
3.	h	**3.**	C
4.	c	**4.**	I
5.	j	**5.**	J
6.	l	**6.**	B
7.	m	**7.**	E
8.	g	**8.**	H
9.	b	**9.**	D
10.	d	**10.**	G
11.	k	**11.**	K
12.	f	**12.**	L
13.	i	**13.**	M
		14.	N
		15.	O
		16.	P
		17.	Q
		18.	R
		19.	S
		20.	T
		21.	U

Activity

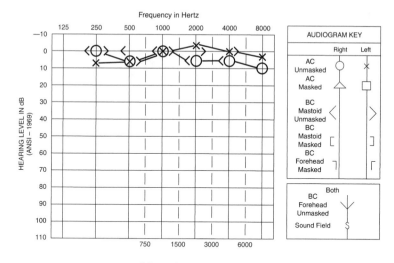

FIGURE 18.5   Normal hearing

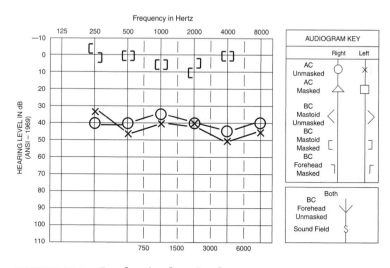

FIGURE 18.6   Conductive hearing loss

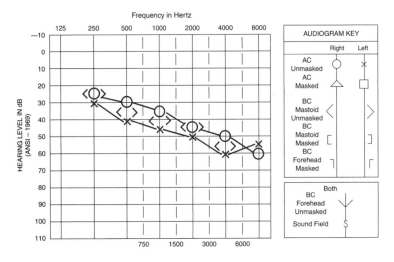

FIGURE 18.7   Sensorineural hearing loss

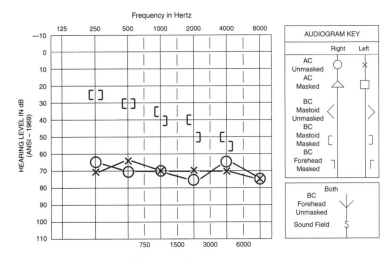

FIGURE 18.8   Mixed hearing loss

Multiple Choice

1. b

2. a

3. c

4. c

5. b

6. d

7. c

8. b

9. a

10. a

11. c

12. c

13. d

14. c

SPEECH AUDIOMETRY

BACKGROUND

The hearing impairment inferred from a pure-tone audiogram cannot depict, beyond the grossest generalizations, the degree of disability in speech communication caused by a hearing loss. Because difficulties in hearing and understanding speech evoke the greatest complaints from patients with hearing impairments, it is logical that tests of hearing function should be performed with speech stimuli as well as pure tones. Modern diagnostic audiometers include circuitry for measuring various aspects of receptive speech communication. Using speech audiometry, audiologists set out to answer questions regarding patients' degree of hearing loss for speech; the levels required for their most comfortable and uncomfortable loudness levels; their range of comfortable loudness; and, perhaps most importantly, their ability to recognize and discriminate the sounds of speech. Speech-language pathologists use reported findings of speech audiometric results in both therapy planning and patient and family counseling.

Speech audiometry takes several forms and serves a number of useful purposes. Speech may be delivered by monitored-live voice, tape, or disk recording to a patient via earphones or loudspeakers. Speech audiometry is helpful in the diagnosis of the type and degree of hearing impairment, in the location of site of lesion, in rehabilitative measures such as evaluation of hearing aids, and in determining the reliability of other tests like the pure-tone audiogram.

When speech audiometry was first introduced in the 1940s, the first measurements made were of threshold, following the concepts of pure-tone audiometry. Patients were asked to signal when they could just barely hear speech, even if they could not discriminate the meaning. This is called the speech-detection threshold (SDT) and has limited utility. The SDT is sometimes called the SAT (speech-awareness threshold). Measurements are in dB HL with a reference to normal hearing for speech.

Following the SDT came the concept of the speech-recognition threshold (SRT). This was originally called the speech-reception threshold. SRT is defined as the lowest intensity at which subjects can barely understand (discriminate) speech. An operational definition of SRT is the lowest intensity at which at least half of the presented materials can be repeated correctly. The audiologist who uses monitored-live voice watches a device on the audiometer called a VU (volume units) meter to be certain that the peak energy of all the words is approximately the same. Usual stimuli are spondaic words (spondees), which are two-syllable words with equal stress on both syllables. Spondees are not found in normal English discourse. The intensity of the speech sounds, either live voice or recorded, is raised and lowered until the subject repeats about 50 percent of the words correctly.

SRTs have several distinct advantages. The most notable is that it is an excellent check on the reliability of pure-tone test results. With some exceptions, there should be close agreement between the SRT and the average of the pure-tone thresholds at 500, 1000, and 2000 Hz (called the pure-tone average [PTA]). Variations in the degree of hearing loss at different frequencies can affect this relationship, such as when hearing is significantly better in the low frequencies than in the highs and motivated patients use the cues they get from the vowel sounds of speech to help them discriminate among spondees. In such cases the SRT may be lower (better) than the PTA. Some older patients have difficulty with speech audiometry because they process more slowly and their SRTs may be poorer than their PTAs. Seasoned clinicians expect SRT-PTA agreement but learn to understand when lack of agreement is explainable or should be considered to indicate poor test reliability.

The early audiologists who pioneered speech audiometry decided that threshold measurements do not reveal the difficulties with understanding speech that patients with hearing loss complain about. This led to the development of tests of speech recognition, which are frequently delivered at comfortable listening levels of 30 to 40 dB above the SRT or at predetermined hearing levels such as conversational intensity (45 dB HL) or MCL. These tests are sometimes comprised of sentences but usually employ lists of words said to be phonetically balanced (PB). Tests are usually carried out by preceding each stimulus word with a short carrier phrase, so the patient might hear "Say the word boy," with "boy" being the stimulus word. Fifty words comprise the list, although many audiologists use half lists. At the completion of the test the number of words correctly repeated is multiplied by 2 percent (or 4 percent in the case of half lists) to determine the speech recognition score. For enhanced test comparisons between tests performed on the same patient by different audiologists the use of recorded testing is recommended. Speech recognition measures presented in varying amounts of background noise help to document the communication difficulties a hearing loss presents and the benefits derived from amplification.

Speech audiometry has also been used to determine what has been called the most comfortable loudness level (MCL), which is usually 40 to 50 dB above the SRT for normals, the uncomfortable loudness level (UCL), or threshold of discomfort (TD), and the range of comfortable loudness (RCL), which is the arithmetic difference between the SRT and the UCL. These measures are particularly useful in the fitting of hearing aids.

Most audiologists today would not consider an audiological evaluation complete without several aspects of speech audiometry. While it is often difficult to utilize specific scores in determining the kinds of difficulty patients experience in their receptive speech communication, the measures just described are an integral part of the audiologist's testing.

OBJECTIVES

1. You should know and understand the terms in the matching exercise.

2. You should be able to fill in the outline, selecting items from the list provided.

3. You should be able to label the different parts of Figure 19.1, showing the performance-intensity functions of speech stimuli.

4. You should be able to predict, within reason, speech test results from an audiogram.

5. You should be able to answer the multiple-choice questions and understand the uses and interpretations of speech audiometry.

6. You should know and understand the terms in the vocabulary list and be able to describe or define each term.

MATCHING

Match the term from the column on the right with its definition.

Definition

1. ___ The SPL at which speech becomes uncomfortably loud

2. ___ Introduction of speech through a microphone during speech audiometry

3. ___ A closed-message word-recognition test with emphasis on unvoiced consonants

4. ___ The highest word-recognition score obtainable from an individual regardless of sensation level

5. ___ The lowest level at which an individual can detect the presence of speech and recognize it as speech

6. ___ Monosyllabic words containing three phonemes each that are used in word-recognition tests

7. ___ A short phrase that precedes the stimulus word during speech audiometry

8. ___ A test that uses pictures to determine word recognition scores for children

9. ___ The difference (in decibels) between the threshold for speech and the level at which speech becomes uncomfortably loud

10. ___ Rapidly delivered, monotonous, and unemotional speech

11. ___ A device used for measurement of speech-recognition thresholds and speech-recognition scores

12. ___ A two-syllable word, used in speech audiometry, that has equal stress on both syllables

13. ___ A graph showing the percentage correct on speech-recognition tests as a function of intensity

14. ___ A list of monosyllabic words used for determination of speech-recognition scores

15. ___ PB Max – PB Min/PB Max

16. ___ The lowest intensity at which 50 percent of a list of spondees can be recognized

17. ___ The intensity (in dB HL) at which speech is judged to be most comfortably loud

18. ___ A closed-set word recognition test

Term

a.   California consonant test

b.   Carrier phrase

c.   Cold running speech

d.   CNC words

e.   Diagnostic audiometer

f.   Monitored-live voice

g.   Most comfortable loudness

h.   PB max

i.   PI function

j.   PB word list

k.   Range of comfortable loudness

l.   Rhyme test

m.   Rollover ratio

n.   Speech-detection threshold

o.   Speech-recognition threshold

p.   Spondaic word

q.   Uncomfortable loudness level

r.   WIPI test

OUTLINE

Speech Audiometry

Speech-Detection Threshold

Purpose

   1. ___

Material

   2. ___

Speech-Recognition Threshold

Purposes

   3. ___

   4. ___

   5. ___

   6. ___

Materials

   7. ___

   8. ___

Speech-Recognition Scores

Purposes

   9. ___

   10. ___

   11. ___

Materials

   12. ___

   13. ___

   14. ___

   15. ___

   16. ___

   17. ___

   18. ___

Select From

A. CNC words

B. California Consonant Test

C. Cold running speech

D. Degree of hearing loss for speech

E. Detect presence of speech

F. Intensity of greatest ease of listening

G. Intensity at which speech is just too loud

H. PB word lists

I. A reference level for SRS

J. Rhyme tests

K. Sentence tests

L. Site-of-lesion diagnosis

M. Spondaic words

N. Synthetic sentence identification

O. Verify audiogram

P. Verify hearing aids' benefit

Q. WIPI test

R. Speech recognition ability

S. 50 percent discrimination of speech

Most Comfortable Loudness	*Uncomfortable Loudness*
Purpose	Purpose
19. ___	**21.** ___
Material	Material
20. ___	**22.** ___

ACTIVITY

Label the four curves shown in Figure 19.1 that illustrate performance intensity functions. Select the terms from the list provided.

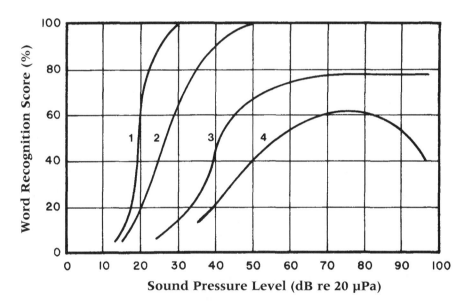

FIGURE 19.1   Performance-intensity functions

Label

1. ___

2. ___

3. ___

4. ___

Term

A. Normal PB curve

B. Normal spondee curve

C. Rollover

D. Speech-recognition loss

MULTIPLE CHOICE

Answer questions 1–7 based on the information contained in the audiogram in Figure 19.2. If you are uncertain of the answer to question 1, check the answer at the end of this unit before proceeding with the questions.

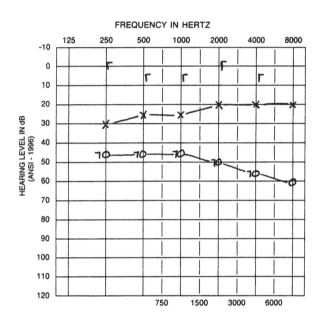

FIGURE 19.2   An audiogram

1. The audiogram illustrates
   a. left mild conductive, right moderate conductive
   b. left mild sensorineural, right moderate sensorineural
   c. left mild conductive, right moderate sensorineural
   d. left moderate sensorineural, right mild conductive

2. A predicted SRT for the left ear is ___ dB HL
   a. 5   c.   45
   b. 25   d.   70

3. A predicted SRS for the left ear is ___ percent
   a. 6   c.   80
   b. 40   d.   100

4. A predicted MCL for the right ear is ___ dB HL
   a. 10   c.   50
   b. 30   d.   80

5. A predicted SRS for the right ear is ___ percent
   a. 10   c.   80
   b. 30   d.   100

6. A predicted UCL for the left ear is ___ dB HL

   a. 5   **c.**   80
   b. 65   **d.**   110

7. A predicted RCL (dynamic range) for the right ear is ___ dB

   a. 0   **c.**   45
   b. 15   **d.**   110

8. The relationship between SRT and SDT is usually

   a. SRT 10 dB lower (better) than SDT
   b. SRT 10 dB higher (poorer) than SDT
   c. SRT the same as SDT
   d. no relationship exists

9. Speech-recognition scores are most commonly determined by using

   a. spondees
   b. PB word lists
   c. cold running speech
   d. WIPI

10. SRTs are usually measured with

   a. PB word lists
   b. spondaic words
   c. rhyming words
   d. nonsense words

11. The PI function for spondees is usually

   a. the same as for PBs
   b. more gradual than for PBs
   c. steeper than for PBs
   d. unreliable above 80 dB HL

12. The last word of the carrier phrase in speech-recognition testing with PB word lists should

   a. strike zero on the volume units (VU) meter
   b. be equal in energy to the PB word
   c. be less intense than the PB word
   d. be more intense than the PB word

13. In audiograms showing sharply falling (in the higher frequencies) sensorineural hearing loss, the SRT is best predicted by the average of the thresholds at ___ Hz

   a. 500 and 1000
   b. 500, 1000, and 2000
   c. 500, 1000, 2000, and 3000
   d. 500, 1000, 2000, 3000, and 4000

14. The speech-recognition score expected of a patient with a mild cochlear hearing loss is ___ percent

    a. 0   **c.** 80

    b. 50   **d.** 100

15. The speech-recognition score expected of a patient with moderate conductive hearing loss is ___ percent

    a. 0   **c.** 70

    b. 50   **d.** 100

16. RCL(DR) is determined by the difference (in decibels) between

    a. UCL and SRT

    b. UCL and MCL

    c. MCL and SRT

    d. UCL and PTA

17. The slope of the normal PI-PB function averages ___ percent per dB

    a. $2\frac{1}{2}$ **c.** 10

    b. 5   **d.** $12\frac{1}{2}$

18. PB Max – PB Min/PB Max is the formula for

    a. percentage of hearing impairment

    b. rollover ratio

    c. word recognition score

    d. none of the above

VOCABULARY

California consonant test

carrier phrase

cold running speech

consonant-nucleus-consonant (CNC) words

dynamic range (DR)

monitored-live voice (MLV)

most comfortable loudness (MCL)

PB Max

performance intensity (P-I) function

phonetically balanced (PB) word lists

range of comfortable loudness (RCL)

rhyme test

rollover ratio

speech audiometer

speech-detection threshold (SDT)

speech-reception threshold (SRT)

speech-recognition score (SRS)

spondaic word (spondee)

spondee threshold (ST)

threshold of discomfort (TD)

uncomfortable loudness level (UCL)

word intelligibility by picture identification (WIPI)

word-recognition score (WRS)

ANSWERS

Matching	*Outline*	*Activity*	*Multiple Choice*
1. q	**1.** E	**1.** B	**1.** c
2. f	**2.** C	**2.** A	**2.** b
3. a	**3.** D	**3.** D	**3.** d
4. h	**4.** I	**4.** C	**4.** d
5. n	**5.** O		**5.** c
6. d	**6.** S		**6.** d
7. b	**7.** C		**7.** c
8. r	**8.** M		**8.** b
9. k	**9.** L		**9.** b
10. c	**10.** P		**10.** b
11. e	**11.** R		**11.** c
12. p	**12.** A		**12.** a
13. i	**13.** B		**13.** a
14. j	**14.** H		**14.** c
15. m	**15.** J		**15.** d
16. o	**16.** K		**16.** a
17. g	**17.** N		**17.** a
18. l	**18.** Q		**18.** b
	19. F		
	20. C		
	21. G		
	22. C		

TUNING FORK TESTS

BACKGROUND

We test human hearing through both air-conduction and bone-conduction pathways. Any sound that courses through the outer ear, middle ear, inner ear, and beyond is heard by air conduction. It is possible to bypass the outer and middle ears by vibrating the skull mechanically and stimulating the inner ear directly by bone conduction as discussed in Unit 4.

Tests of hearing utilizing tuning forks are by no means modern, but they illustrate hearing via these two pathways. The tuning fork, borrowed from the music profession, vibrates sinusoidally and comes closer to generating a pure tone than any other nonelectronic device. The tuning fork is set into vibration by holding the stem in the hand and striking one of the tines against a firm but resilient surface such as the heel of the shoe. While tuning-fork tests can be useful in differentiating types of hearing loss, they are nonquantifiable, should be used only to verify audiometric data, and must be specified in terms of the frequency of the fork being used.

Conductive hearing loss arises when sound transmission through the air conduction pathway is disrupted. In other words, sound is not conducted into the hearing nerve properly. Conductive hearing losses arise from disorders in either the outer or middle ears. Sounds delivered to the ear via air conduction will be attenuated in the presence of outer- or middle-ear disorders to a degree commensurate with the severity of the disorder. If the sound is delivered to the ear via bone conduction, essentially bypassing the outer and middle ears, the sound will be heard normally, assuming there is no disorder in the sensorineural mechanism (comprised of the inner ear and the neural pathways beyond). A pure sensorineural hearing loss assumes the outer-ear and middle-ear structures are functioning normally. It is an understanding of the air-conduction and bone-conduction pathways that gives rise to an understanding of tuning-fork tests.

The *Schwabach test* compares the hearing sensitivity of a patient with that of the examiner. The tuning fork is set into vibration, and the stem is first pressed against the mastoid process (the bony protrusion behind the ear) of the patient. When the diminishing vibrations are no longer heard, the examiner immediately places the stem of the tuning fork behind his or her own ear and, using a watch, notes the number of seconds that the tone is audible after the patient stops hearing it. A normal Schwabach occurs when the patient and the examiner stop hearing the tone emitted by the fork at approximately the same time. A diminished Schwabach is noted when the examiner hears the tone longer than the patient with the degree of loss being quantified to some degree in seconds. If patients have a conductive hearing loss, bone conduction is normal, and they will hear the tone for at least as long as the examiner, and sometimes longer. Interpretation of test results in cases of mixed hearing losses (combined conductive and sensorineural hearing loss in the same ear) is especially difficult. If there is a difference in sensitivity between the two inner ears, a patient will probably respond to sound heard through the better ear, which can cause a *false normal Schwabach.*

Performance of the *Rinne test* compares patients' hearing sensitivity by bone conduction to their sensitivity by air conduction. They are asked to state whether the tone is louder when the tuning-fork stem is held against the mastoid process or when the tines of the fork that are generating an air-conducted sound are held next to the opening of the ear. Since the air-conduction pathway is more efficient than the bone-conduction pathway, patients with normal hearing and those with sensorineural hearing loss will hear the tone louder at the ear than behind the ear. This is called a positive Rinne. If patients' bone-conduction hearing is better than their air-conduction hearing (a conductive or mixed hearing loss), they will hear a louder tone with the stem of the fork behind the ear. This is called a negative Rinne. Sometimes patients manifest what has been called a *false negative Rinne,* which occurs when the nontest ear responds to the tone by bone conduction, a frequent phenomenon given that the test is typically not done while masking the opposite ear (see Unit 9).

The *Bing test* is performed by placing the tuning-fork stem against the mastoid process behind the ear while alternately opening and closing the patient's ear canal with a finger. When the canal is closed on a person with normal hearing or sensorineural hearing loss, low-frequency bone-conducted signals are heard more loudly, a phenomenon known as the occlusion effect; this is a positive Bing. Patients with conductive hearing loss will not experience this sensation, and the Bing test is said to be negative. As with the Schwabach and Rinne tests, the danger of a response to the tone by the nontest ear is ever present.

The *Weber test* is a test of lateralization and is typically performed with the examiner pressing the stem of the tuning fork against the patient's forehead. The patient simply responds if the tone is heard in the left ear, right ear, both ears, or in the midline. People with normal hearing or with equal amounts of the same type of hearing loss in both ears (conductive, sensorineural, or mixed) will report a midline sensation. Patients with sensorineural hearing loss in one ear will hear the tone in their better ear. Patients with conductive hearing loss in one ear will hear the tone in their poorer ear.

OBJECTIVES

1. You should know and understand the terms in the matching exercise.

2. You should be able to fill in the outline, selecting items from the list provided.

3. You should understand the four tuning-fork tests discussed in this unit in terms of performance and interpretation.

4. You should be able to answer the multiple-choice questions and understand the purpose and use of tuning forks.

5. You should know and understand the terms in the vocabulary list and be able to describe or define each term.

MATCHING

Match the term from the column on the right with its definition.

Definition

1. ___ The perception of increased loudness of a bone-conducted tone when the outer ear is occluded

2. ___ A tuning-fork test that compares the patient's hearing sensitivity by bone conduction with the examiner's

3. ___ Sounds that are conducted to the inner ear by vibration of the bones of the skull

4. ___ Attenuation of sounds as they pass through an abnormality of the outer ear or middle ear

5. ___ A metal instrument with a stem and two tines that is designed to vibrate at a single frequency

6. ___ A tone of only one frequency with no overtones

7. ___ A tuning-fork test that checks for the occlusion effect to determine the presence of conductive loss

8. ___ A tuning-fork test that compares hearing sensitivity presented by bone conduction to air conduction

9. ___ Conduction of sound to the inner ear by way of the outer and middle ear

10. ___ A tuning-fork test to determine whether a bone-conducted tone is heard in the right, left, or both ears

11. ___ Hearing loss produced by abnormality of the inner ear or auditory nerve

Term

a. Air conduction

b. Bing test

c. Bone conduction

d. Conductive hearing loss

e. Occlusion effect

f. Pure tone

g. Rinne test

h. Schwabach test

i. Sensorineural hearing loss

j. Tuning fork

k. Weber test

OUTLINE

Tuning Fork Tests

Rinne

1. ___

2. ___

3. ___

4. ___

5. ___

6. ___

Schwabach

7. ___

8. ___

9. ___

Bing

10. ___

11. ___

12. ___

13. ___

14. ___

Weber

15. ___

16. ___

17. ___

18. ___

Select From

A. Absence of occlusion effect means conductive hearing loss

B. Compares AC sensitivity to BC

C. Compares patient's BC hearing to examiner's

D. Frequency must be specified

E. Heard in better ear in sensorineural hearing loss

F. Heard in poorer ear in conductive hearing loss

G. Louder by AC means normal or sensorineural loss

H. Louder by BC means conductive loss

I. Presence of occlusion effect means normal or sensorineural loss

J. Outer ear is occluded

K. Stem held against forehead

L. Stem held against mastoid

M. Tine held next to ear

ACTIVITY

Using Figure 20.1, indicate the position in which a tuning fork should be held for each test.

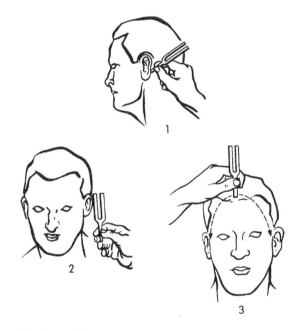

FIGURE 20.1

Label

1. ___

2. ___

3. ___

Term

A. Bing test

B. Rinne test

C. Schwabach test

D. Weber test

MULTIPLE CHOICE

1. One thing that should always be specified when reporting the results of tuning-fork tests is the
   a. frequency of the fork
   b. amplitude of the fork
   c. pressure of the fork against the head
   d. weight of the fork

2. A problem that tuning-fork tests have in common with any measurement made by bone conduction is that
   a. the nontest ear may hear the tone by bone conduction
   b. the patient may feel the vibrations
   c. pressure against the skull is a variable
   d. all of the above

3. In bilateral sensorineural hearing loss, the tuning-fork tests will theoretically show
   a. Bing negative: Rinne negative
   b. Bing positive: Rinne negative
   c. Bing negative: Rinne positive
   d. Bing positive: Rinne positive

4. A patient has a severe sensorineural hearing loss in the left ear and normal hearing in the right ear. Results on the Rinne test would be
   a. left positive: right positive
   b. left false negative: right positive
   c. left negative: right negative
   d. left false negative: right false positive

5. In unilateral conductive hearing loss, the Weber test will result in the sound being heard in the
   a. better ear
   b. both ears
   c. poorer ear
   d. neither ear

6. A normal Schwabach can mean
   a. normal hearing or conductive hearing loss
   b. normal hearing or sensorineural hearing loss
   c. normal hearing or mixed hearing loss
   d. sensorineural hearing loss

The next three questions are based on the proposition that your patient has a moderate conductive hearing loss in the left ear and a moderate sensorineural hearing loss in the right ear.

7. Results on the Rinne test should be
   a. positive right: positive left
   b. negative right: negative left
   c. positive right: negative left
   d. false negative right: negative left

8. If masking is used in the nontest ear, results on the Schwabach should be
   a. normal right: normal left
   b. diminished right: prolonged left
   c. prolonged right: diminished left
   d. normal right: diminished left

9. Results on the Bing test should be
   a. positive right: positive left
   b. negative right: negative left
   c. positive right: negative left
   d. negative right: positive left

VOCABULARY

air conduction (AC)	pure tone
Bing test	Rinne test
bone conduction (BC)	Schwabach test
conductive hearing loss	sensorineural hearing loss
lateralization	tuning fork
occlusion effect (OE)	Weber test

ANSWERS

Matching	Outline	Activity	Multiple Choice
1. e	1. B	1. A, B, C	1. a
2. h	2. D	2. B	2. d
3. c	3. G	3. D	3. d
4. d	4. H		4. b
5. j	5. L		5. c
6. f	6. M		6. a
7. b	7. C		7. d
8. g	8. D		8. b
9. a	9. L		9. c
10. k	10. A		
11. i	11. D		
	12. I		
	13. J		
	14. L		
	15. D		
	16. E		
	17. F		
	18. K		

CASE STUDIES

HISTORY

Your patient is a 26-year-old female with a complaint of diminished hearing for several years "that seems to be getting worse." Her mother has told you that the patient experienced ear infections as a small child, but the patient herself has no memory of this. She has increased difficulty hearing while chewing but seems, to her surprise, to understand speech better in a noisy background than in quiet places. The patient has two older sisters with hearing losses that began in early adulthood. One wears hearing aids successfully and the other was helped by surgery, the nature of which the patient does not know. She, along with members of her family, has a bluish cast to the whites of her eyes. Given the audiometric data on the following page and this history, make your diagnosis and substantiate it.

DIAGNOSIS

Type of Loss Right: _____ Left: _____

Probable Etiology

_____

_____

Case Management

_____

_____

_____

_____

Reasons for Decision

_____

_____

_____

_____

AUDIOMETRIC DATA

Test	Right Ear	Left Ear
SRT	25 dB HL	35 dB HL
SRS	98%	100%
ARTs (ipsilateral)	Absent	Absent
ARTs (contralateral)	Absent	Absent
Static compliance	0.7 cc	0.65 cc
ABR	All waves prolonged; interpeak latencies normal; latency-intensity function normal	All waves prolonged; interpeak latencies normal; latency-intensity function normal
TEOAE	Absent	Absent
Tone decay test	0 dB of decay in 60 seconds	5 dB of decay in 60 seconds

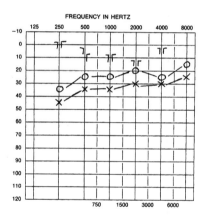

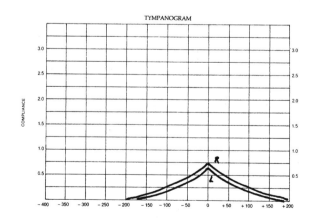

CORRECT DIAGNOSIS

Type of Loss

Right: Conductive
Left: Conductive

Probable Etiology

Bilateral otosclerosis

Case Management

Refer to an otologist with a good track record doing stapedectomies. Include all audiometric data and a report stating your suspicions. Request a letter to learn the otologic diagnosis and proposed treatment.

Reasons for Decision

The normal bone conduction, air-bone gaps, and excellent speech recognition scores all indicate a conductive hearing loss. The tympanograms are Type A in both ears, and crossed and uncrossed acoustic reflexes are absent at the limits of the equipment, suggesting middle-ear disorders. Static compliance is normal and does not assist in diagnosis. The low-frequency tilt of the audiogram suggests stiffness in the middle-ear system. The Carhart notch suggests otosclerosis, along with the family history of females with progressive hearing loss, blue sclera, paracusis willisii, and deprecusis. All special tests are consistent with a conductive hearing loss. The infections as a child have no bearing because the hearing loss had its onset years after the infections had ceased. Because one sister was helped by surgery and the other did well with hearing aids (suggesting good speech recognition ability), it is likely that they too have otosclerosis.

HISTORY

Your patient is a 39-year-old male with a history of sudden hearing loss in the right ear and vertigo. Previous to an incident several months earlier, the patient had no difficulty with either hearing or balance. The course of symptoms is described as follows: The patient first noted a sensation of fullness in his right ear along with some slight difficulty understanding through that ear over the telephone. On the second day he noticed a humming noise in that ear followed by a loud roaring sound. He suddenly had the sensation of whirling and was unable to keep his balance; he became ill and vomited several times. He now feels that he has no hearing in his right ear although the spinning sensation has completely disappeared. Both his parents had difficulty hearing when they became much older. His greatest communication difficulty is in group situations or when people speak softly to him on his right side. Given the audiometric findings on the following page and this history, make your diagnosis and substantiate it.

DIAGNOSIS

Type of Loss Right: _____ Left: _____

Probable Etiology

_____

_____

Case Management

_____

_____

_____

_____

Reasons for Decision

_____

_____

_____

_____

AUDIOMETRIC DATA

Test	Right Ear	Left Ear
SRT	70 dB HL	5 dB HL
SRS	34%	100%
ARTs (ipsilateral)	100 dB HL	90 dB HL
ARTs (contralateral)	100 dB HL	90 dB HL
Static compliance	0.9 cc	0.65 cc
ABR	All waves prolonged; interpeak latencies normal; latency-intensity function for wave V steep	All waves normal; interpeak latencies normal; latency-intensity function for wave V normal
TEOAE	Absent	Present
Tone decay test	15 dB of decay in 60 seconds	5 dB of decay in 60 seconds

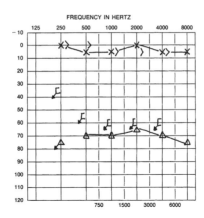

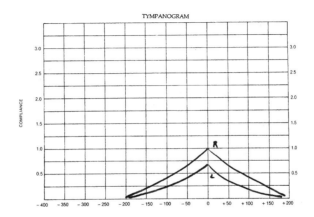

CORRECT DIAGNOSIS

Type of Loss

Right: Sensorineural (Cochlear)
Left: Normal hearing

Probable Etiology

Unilateral Ménière disease

Case Management

Refer to an otologist with comments on your suspicions and recommend electronystagmography. If you can perform ENG in your clinic, proceed with the test following your clinic's protocol. Request a report from the physician and arrange for the patient to return for further counseling and longitudinal testing to monitor for fluctuation or progression.

Reasons for Decision

The roaring tinnitus and full aural sensations are part of the usual prodroma of Ménière disease, probably caused by increased endolymphatic pressure. All of the special tests suggest a cochlear site of lesion. The speech-recognition score is extremely poor in the right ear. All tests in the right ear should have been performed with masking in the left ear. The presence of acoustic reflexes at normal hearing levels (low sensation levels in the right ear), along with the steep ABR latency-intensity function and absent TEOAEs suggests a cochlear disorder. The hearing losses experienced by the patient's parents do not bear on the diagnosis because they are probably caused by aging. The difficulty hearing in groups is typical of severe unilateral losses. Because hearing is normal in the left ear, the patient relies on it and is unaware of the residual hearing in the right ear.

HISTORY

Your patient is a 34-month-old male who is brought to you by his parents. They are not certain whether a hearing loss is present, although the child says "huh" a good deal. The father believes that he "does not pay attention." The child has been "slightly behind" his two older, normal siblings (a boy and a girl) in his language development milestones. A pediatrician has treated the child with antibiotics for "ear infections" on a few occasions, but more often for "tonsillitis." No marked temperature elevations were associated with these episodes, and the child is otherwise healthy. There is no family history of hearing loss, although his father has difficulty understanding speech in groups and has a constant high-pitched tinnitus since serving two years in the artillery. The child tired quickly before all the desired hearing tests could be completed, but given the history and the limited audiometric data on the following page, make your diagnosis and substantiate it.

DIAGNOSIS

Type of Loss Right: _____ Left: _____

Probable Etiology

_____

_____

Case Management

_____

_____

_____

_____

Reasons for Decision

_____

_____

_____

_____

AUDIOMETRIC DATA

Test	Right Ear	Left Ear
SRT	20 dB HL	25 dB HL
SRS	?	?
ARTs (ipsilateral)	Absent	Absent
ARTs (contralateral)	Absent	Absent
Static compliance	0.25 cc	0.20 cc
ABR	All waves prolonged; interpeak latencies normal; latency-intensity function normal	All waves prolonged; interpeak latencies normal; latency-intensity function normal
TEOAE	Absent	Absent

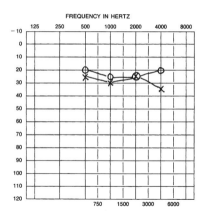

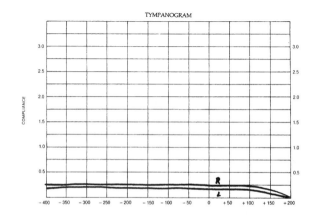

CORRECT DIAGNOSIS

Type of Loss

Right: Conductive
Left: Conductive

Probable Etiology

Bilateral serous effusion

Case Management

Refer to an otologist with all your findings and suspicions. Make an appointment for further audiometric study, especially bone conduction. Request a report of the physician's findings. Stress to the parents the importance of a complete audiometric examination after all medical and/or surgical treatment has been completed. If hearing is normal upon the return visit, consider referring to a speech-language pathologist to test for language delay secondary to sensory deprivation. Suggest that the father consider a hearing evaluation for a diagnosis of his hearing problem.

Reasons for Decision

The agreement between the SRT and pure-tone average makes the diagnosis of mild hearing loss likely. The fact that the child did not take the bone-conduction test and the lack of speech-recognition scores makes it impossible to state with certainty that the hearing loss is purely conductive (hence the need for further testing); however, the Type B tympanograms, the absent acoustic reflexes, low static compliance, and flat audiometric configuration all suggest fluid in the middle ear. Because there was no ear drainage, pain, or fever in the history, it is more likely that the hearing loss is due to serous effusion than to active infection. This, of course, must be determined medically. The father's hearing loss is acquired, probably because of noise, and is irrelevant to the diagnosis of the child's problem.

HISTORY

Your patient is a 23-year-old male who was referred by his attorney for routine hearing tests because of a gradual hearing loss in his left ear associated with noise. The patient is a construction worker. There is no history of ear infections, vertigo, or tinnitus and no reported family members with hearing loss. The patient claims that he is "totally deaf" in the left ear and requests that you write a letter to this effect "to whom it may concern." He claims that he cannot hear people speak at all when they are on his left side. Given the history and the audiometric data on the following page make your diagnosis and substantiate it.

DIAGNOSIS

Type of Loss Right: _____ Left: _____

Probable Etiology

_____

_____

Case Management

_____

_____

_____

_____

Reasons for Decision

_____

_____

_____

_____

AUDIOMETRIC DATA

Test	Right Ear	Left Ear
SRT	5 dB HL	NR
SRS	100%	NR
ARTs (ipsilateral)	95 dB HL	95 dB HL
ARTs (contralateral)	100 dB HL	95 dB HL
Static compliance	0.62 cc	0.66 cc
ABR	All waves normal; interpeak latencies normal; latency-intensity function normal	All waves normal; interpeak latencies normal; latency-intensity function normal
TEOAE	Present	Present

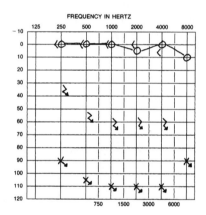

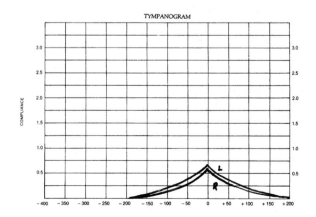

CORRECT DIAGNOSIS

Type of Loss

Right: Normal hearing
Left: Normal hearing

Probable Etiology

Nonorganic hearing loss (probably malingering)

CASE MANAGEMENT

Prepare a report in detail outlining your reasons for suspecting nonorganic hearing loss and the tests that support the diagnosis. Retain and carefully file all test forms or paper readouts for easy retrieval. Explain to the patient that his test results are inconsistent but that you believe the hearing in his left ear to be normal or near normal. Write a letter to his attorney stating the same thing. Do not use the word "malingering." Suggest reevaluation.

Reasons for Decision

Your suspicions are aroused when the patient claims that he cannot hear people "at all" from the left side. The first audiometric tip-off to nonorganicity was the obvious lack of a shadow curve on the audiogram. If the left ear truly had a total loss, the air-conduction and speech recognition thresholds would have been about 55 dB (average interaural attenuation) and the bone-conduction thresholds no worse than about 15 dB. Unmasked speech recognition scores obtained at high levels in the "deaf" ear should approach 100 percent as the opposite (normal) ear should respond. The normal levels at which acoustic reflexes were elicited with stimulation to the left ear prove that a total hearing loss is impossible. The Stenger test's minimum contralateral interference level of 35 dB in the left ear shows that the tone was heard loud enough at that level to make a tone in the right ear at 10 dB inaudible. Further special tests should have been performed as time allowed. High on the list of desirable tests would be the Stenger, using spondaic words and several different frequencies; the pure-tone DAF; and the SPAR test. Existing evidence for nonorganic hearing loss is clear, and malingering is likely because of the involvement of an attorney and potential lawsuit, but psychogenesis cannot be ruled out with certainty. If the hearing loss was truly caused by noise, it would have been less severe and bilateral in nature. Remember that you cannot legally release your findings or impressions to another party without express written permission by the patient.

HISTORY

Your patient is a 42-year-old right-handed male who complains of a high-pitched ringing in his ears, which is louder and more prolonged after noise exposure than had formerly been the case. He is fond of deer and duck hunting and enjoys listening to rock music under earphones. His two sisters have progressive hearing losses that began in their twenties and seemed to get worse during pregnancy. The patient is uncertain whether he has a hearing loss per se but notices that speech often sounds muffled, and he has difficulty hearing in groups or in background noise. He has never had ear infections. Given the history and the audiometric data on the following page make your diagnosis and substantiate it.

DIAGNOSIS

Type of Loss Right: _____ Left: _____

Probable Etiology

_____

_____

Case Management

_____

_____

_____

_____

Reasons for Decision

_____

_____

_____

_____

AUDIOMETRIC DATA

Test	Right Ear	Left Ear
SRT	15 dB HL	25 dB HL
SRS	100%	100%
ART at 1000 Hz (ipsilateral)	85 dB HL	90 dB HL
ARTs (contralateral)	95 dB HL	90 dB HL
Static compliance	0.52 cc	0.70 cc
ABR	All waves prolonged; interpeak latencies normal; latency-intensity function steep	All waves prolonged; interpeak latencies normal; latency-intensity function steep
TEOAE	Absent	Absent
Tone decay test at 4000 Hz	5 dB of decay in 60 seconds	5 dB of decay in 60 seconds

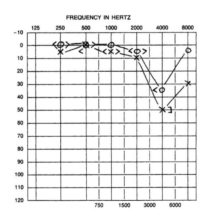

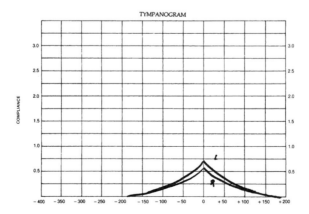

CORRECT DIAGNOSIS

Type of Loss

Right: Sensorineural (cochlear)
Left: Sensorineural (cochlear)

Probable Etiology

Exposure to high noise levels

Case Management

Explain to the patient the nature of the loss and why the cause is probably noise. Encourage abstention from or minimizing exposure to noise. Suggest the use of hearing protectors, possibly in the form of special impact-noise plugs. If possible, fit the plugs yourself and/or provide the patient with precise information on where foam plugs can be obtained and their approximate cost. Encourage lower levels when listening to music and the use of loudspeakers rather than earphones. Arrange for reevaluation of hearing in six months and stress the importance of checking for progression of the loss. Interoctave frequencies (3000 and 6000 Hz) should have been tested because of the greater than 20 dB differences in thresholds at octave points.

Reasons for Decision

The audiogram shows the typical acoustic trauma notch; note that the loss at 4000 Hz is greater in the left ear, which is typical of persons firing a rifle from the right shoulder. The family history sounds like otosclerosis, although you cannot be certain of that, and it is unrelated to the patient's problem. It is likely that the patient experiences some increased loss of hearing and tinnitus immediately after noise exposure, both of which had been recovering to a greater extent in the past until the threshold shifts became more permanent. It is also likely that the patient himself realizes that noise is a probable cause of his difficulty, based on his own subjective impressions and his history.

HISTORY

Your patient is a 16-year-old female with a lifelong history of ear infections. She reports having had mastoidectomies on both sides. A strong pungent odor is noticeable near her ears. There is no family history of hearing loss. She claims that her hearing fluctuates, at times appearing to be near normal and at other times creating severe problems in communication. She has tried a hearing aid in her right ear but constant drainage made its use impossible. She has since lost the aid. Her family doctor has told her that nothing can be done to improve her hearing and has her on a renewable prescription for eardrops. Given the case history and the audiometric data on the following page, make your diagnosis and substantiate it.

DIAGNOSIS

Type of Loss Right: _____ Left: _____

Probable Etiology

_____

_____

Case Management

_____

_____

_____

_____

Reasons for Decision

_____

_____

_____

_____

AUDIOMETRIC DATA

Test	Right Ear	Left Ear
SRT	45 dB HL	40 dB HL
SRS	92%	94%
ARTs (ipsilateral)	Untestable	Untestable
ARTs (contralateral)	Untestable	Untestable
Static compliance	No seal	No seal
ABR	All waves prolonged; interpeak latencies normal; latency-intensity function normal	All waves prolonged; interpeak latencies normal; latency-intensity function normal
TEOAE	Absent	Absent
Tone decay test at 4000 Hz	0 dB of decay in 60 seconds	5 dB of decay in 60 seconds

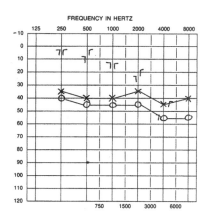

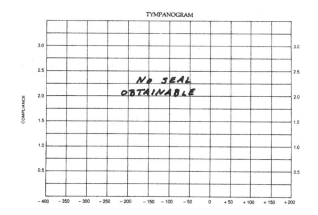

CORRECT DIAGNOSIS

Type of Loss

Right: Mixed
Left: Mixed

Probable Etiology

Chronic otitis media

Case Management

Discuss with the patient the type of hearing loss she has and its relationship to her history of infections and strongly suggest that she consider a second opinion by an otologist. Provide a detailed report to the otologist and request a letter with his or her diagnosis and plan for therapy. Discuss the possibility of hearing aids if there is no evidence that treatment will result in improvement in hearing. Obtain written medical clearance before proceeding with a hearing aid evaluation and, if the ear drainage is a persistent problem, consider a bone-conduction aid. Arrange for periodic monitoring of the hearing loss and keep the patient informed of her progress. See that the patient understands the implications of the sensorineural portion of her hearing loss and recognizes that, although her hearing may be improved considerably, it cannot be made completely normal.

Reasons for Decision

The air-bone gap, high speech-recognition scores, and drop in bone-conduction sensitivity in the high frequencies all indicate a mixed loss that is predominantly conductive. The cochlear reserve may actually be better than the bone-conduction thresholds indicate because of alterations in the inertial mode of bone conduction caused by the middle-ear disorder. The inability to obtain a seal upon immittance testing and the large c_1 values suggest tympanic membrane perforations, which should have been visible upon otoscopic examination prior to testing. The strong odor at the ears suggests the possibility of cholesteatomas. Diplomacy is necessary in making the new referral so that your comments will not be construed as critical of the family doctor, although surely this consultation may be necessary.

HISTORY

Your patient is a 51-year-old male who complains of vague difficulty in understanding speech, especially in noisy or otherwise untoward listening circumstances. He has no history of ear disease, skull trauma, balance difficulties, or noise exposure. Sometimes he feels that his understanding is improved if he pays very close attention. He has been seen for medical examination and no explanation for his difficulty was offered, although you are not certain of the extent of this examination. Given the history and the audiometric data on the following page, make your diagnosis and substantiate it.

DIAGNOSIS

Type of Loss Right: _____ Left: _____

Probable Etiology

_____

_____

Case Management

_____

_____

_____

_____

Reasons for Decision

_____

_____

_____

_____

AUDIOMETRIC DATA

Test	Right Ear	Left Ear
SRT	0 dB HL	5 dB HL
SRS	98%	100%
ARTs (ipsilateral)	85 dB HL	90 dB HL
ARTs (contralateral)	Absent	Absent
Static compliance	0.72 cc	0.80 cc
ABR	All waves normal; interpeak latencies normal; latency-intensity function normal	All waves normal; interpeak latencies normal; latency-intensity function normal
TEOAE	Present	Present
Tone decay test at 4000 Hz	0 dB of decay in 60 seconds	5 dB of decay in 60 seconds

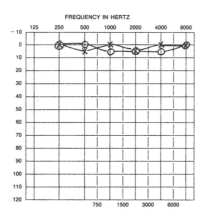

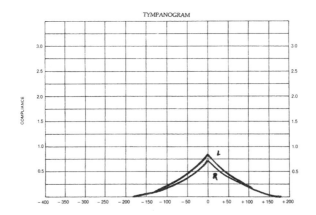

CORRECT DIAGNOSIS

Type of Loss

Right: Normal sensitivity
Left: Normal sensitivity

Probable Etiology

Unknown; possible brain stem lesion

Case Management

Reschedule the patient for a complete battery of special tests for central auditory disorders to include AMLR, PI-PB functions, SSI-ICM, SSI-CCM, staggered spondaic words, and others available. Tell the patient that his difficulty is not in sounds being loud enough because the audiogram indicates normal hearing for pure tones. Explain that additional stress will have to be placed on his speech recognition ability to determine the extent of his difficulty beyond what can be derived from testing with standard word lists. Discuss referral to a neurologist, which would best be done after additional audiometric studies have been completed.

Reasons for Decision

The normal hearing sensitivity, with the kinds of complaints the patient makes, alerts you to a possible central disorder. Present ipsilateral acoustic reflexes at normal levels indicate normal middle ears and acoustic pathways, including VIIth nerve integrity, short of the crossover pathways in the brain stem. Absent contralateral acoustic reflexes suggest that the crossover pathways are involved. More definitive testing should help in the diagnosis, but a neurological referral is imperative in any case.

HISTORY

Your patient is a 19-year-old female college student. Her main complaint is a hearing loss that presents more difficulty in hearing and understanding speech than in hearing environmental sounds. She has had this difficulty as long as she can remember and does not believe it is getting worse. There are no known family members with a hearing loss, and she has never had any ear infections, nor has she worn hearing aids. The patient's speech is quite intelligible but there is some distortion in the production of her sibilant sounds, and her vocal tone is rather monotonous. She managed to get good grades in high school, but now that she is in college she finds school much more difficult and believes it is because of her hearing problem. You notice that she speaks rather loudly. Given the history and the audiometric data on the following page make your diagnosis and substantiate it.

DIAGNOSIS

Type of Loss Right: _____   Left: _____

Probable Etiology

_____

_____

Case Management

_____

_____

_____

_____

Reasons for Decision

_____

_____

_____

_____

AUDIOMETRIC DATA

Test	Right Ear	Left Ear
SRT	45 dB HL	40 dB HL
SRS	86%	82%
ARTs (ipsilateral)	90 dB HL	95 dB HL
ARTs (contralateral)	90 dB HL	90 dB HL
Static compliance	0.80 cc	0.78 cc
ABR	All waves prolonged; interpeak latencies normal; latency-intensity function steep	All waves prolonged; interpeak latencies normal; latency-intensity function steep
TEOAE	Absent	Absent
Tone decay test at 4000 Hz	10 dB of decay in 60 seconds	15 dB of decay in 60 second

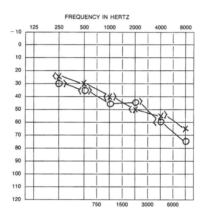

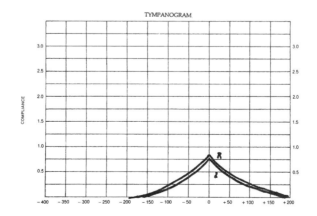

CORRECT DIAGNOSIS

Type of Loss

Right: Sensorineural (probably cochlear)
Left: Sensorineural (probably cochlear)

Probable Etiology

Unknown; possibly congenital

Case Management

Discuss with the patient the possibility of a hearing aid evaluation, adjustment period with hearing aids, and a period of auditory rehabilitation and hearing aid orientation. Ascertain that the patient understands the nature of her hearing loss. Arrange for medical consultation prior to making ear impressions, if this is required in your state. Try to make a positive yet realistic appraisal of the patient's potential for hearing aid use. If she wishes medical consultation on the irreversibility of her hearing loss, offer to provide your findings to the physician of her choice. Check with the physician on possible blood studies and inquire about her interest in genetic counseling. If she is not interested in audiological rehabilitation at this time, recommend that she have annual reevaluations of her hearing.

Reasons for Decision

The absent air-bone gaps and diminished speech-recognition scores, along with the normal tympanograms, indicate sensorineural hearing loss. The low sensation level acoustic reflexes absent OAEs and ABR results are consistent with a cochlear site of lesion. There is simply not enough information in the history to hazard more than a guess about the cause of the loss. The fact that the patient does not know of family members with hereditary hearing loss does not mean that there have been none. The loss may also have been acquired at an early age, caused by some disease.

HISTORY

Your patient is a 58-year-old female with a complaint of hearing loss in her right ear. The difficulty was first noticed about five years earlier and has been gradually progressive to the point where she relies entirely on her left ear for communication. She does not experience true vertigo, but frequently she has attacks of unsteadiness and occasional headaches. She also complains of a constant noise in her right ear, which she describes as "bacon frying." Her family physician has told her that the hearing loss is related to several episodes of middle-ear infection that she had as a child. Her main communication problem is in groups or noisy backgrounds, which she attempts to avoid. Given this history and the audiometric data on the following page, make your diagnosis and substantiate it.

DIAGNOSIS

Type of Loss Right: _____ Left: _____

Probable Etiology

_____

_____

Case Management

_____

_____

_____

_____

Reasons for Decision

_____

_____

_____

_____

AUDIOMETRIC DATA

Test	Right Ear	Left Ear
SRT	50 dB HL	5 dB HL
SRS	6%	100%
ARTs (ipsilateral)	Absent	85 dB HL
ARTs (contralateral)	Absent	80 dB HL
Static compliance	0.80 cc	0.83 cc
ABR	All waves prolonged after Wave I; Wave I to III latency increased; latency-intensity function shallow	All waves normal; interpeak latencies normal; latency-intensity function normal
TEOAE	Present	Present
Tone-decay test	30+ dB of decay in 60 seconds	5 dB of decay in 60 seconds

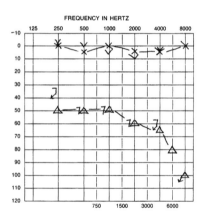

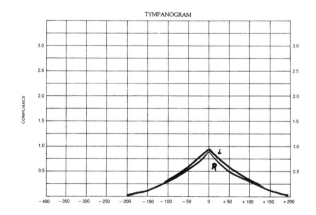

CORRECT DIAGNOSIS

Type of Loss

Right: Sensorineural (probably neural)
Left: Normal

Probable Etiology

Acoustic neuroma—right side

Case Management

Make a prompt referral, if possible to a neuro-otologist or to an otologist with experience in dealing with neural lesions in the auditory tract. Detail all your findings and advise him or her that the history and auditory findings are consistent with a possible retrocochlear lesion. You may discuss your impressions of a possible lesion of the VIIIth nerve with the patient, but should hesitate to put it into a report that is leaving your clinic. Short of frightening the patient, do all you can to see that the referral is followed through. Request that the physician send you results of his or her diagnostic tests (e.g., ENG and radiologic studies), along with the diagnosis and proposed treatment.

Reasons for Decision

The left ear is completely normal on all tests and the right ear shows a moderate loss by both air and bone conduction. SRTs agree nicely with the pure-tone averages, but the speech-recognition scores are extremely poor in the right ear for a moderate loss and first raise suspicions of a retrocochlear lesion. The tinnitus is also not of the usual variety described by patients with cochlear pathology. Abnormal ABRs, present TEOAEs and marked tone decay all fit with a neural lesion in the right ear. The gradual progressive nature of the loss, the type of dizziness, and the headaches all call for an immediate referral to confirm or deny the presence of a space-occupying lesion. The history of ear infections is unrelated to the present hearing loss.

HISTORY

Your patient is an 82-year-old man with a history of gradually progressive hearing loss in both ears over the past fifteen years. He is brought, reluctantly, to the clinic by his daughter-in-law, who complains privately that "he does not pay attention." He claims that sometimes he hears better than at other times and compliments you on the fact that you are easier to understand than most people. He has tried several hearing aids, which were useless to him; he has no desire to purchase any more hearing aids. Because he finds listening in groups difficult, he has ceased attending church, parties, and the theater. He claims that people do not speak clearly and that he understands better when they speak more slowly. Given the history and the audiometric data on the following page, make your diagnosis and substantiate it.

DIAGNOSIS

Type of Loss Right: _____ Left: _____

Probable Etiology

_____

_____

Case Management

_____

_____

_____

_____

Reasons for Decision

_____

_____

_____

_____

AUDIOMETRIC DATA

Test	Right Ear	Left Ear
SRT	50 dB HL	45 dB HL
SRS	62%	58%
ART at 1000 Hz (ipsilateral)	95 dB HL	95 dB HL
ART at 2000 Hz (contralateral)	90 dB HL	100 dB HL
Static compliance	0.92 cc	0.65 cc
ABR	All waves normal at high SLs; interpeak latencies normal; latency-intensity function steep	All waves normal at high SLs; interpeak latencies normal; latency-intensity function steep
TEOAE	Absent	Absent
Tone-decay test	10 dB of decay in 60 seconds	15 dB of decay in 60 seconds

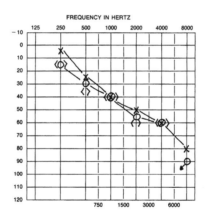

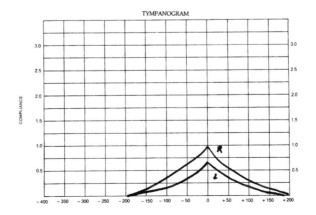

CORRECT DIAGNOSIS

Type of Loss

Right: Sensorineural
Left: Sensorineural

Probable Etiology

Presbycusis

Case Management

Discuss the possibility of amplification for a trial period. In counseling the family, make sure that you speak directly to the patient, although the daughter-in-law should be present. Listen carefully to his complaints and do not provide more information on the nature of the hearing loss than the patient seems to desire. Advise the family that given the patient's past experiences, hearing aids should be purchased on a trial basis until it has been demonstrated that they are of value, and that this cannot really be achieved unless the patient enrolls for a period of auditory rehabilitation that emphasizes coping strategies. Suggest the possibility of assistive listening devices, such as a personal FM system and telephone amplifier. Be as reassuring as possible, short of making an unethical guarantee that the hearing loss will not progress significantly. Arrange for periodic reevaluations and, if the patient agrees, for earmold fabrication. If state law requires medical concurrence before proceeding, explain this to the family and assist in the arrangements.

Reasons for Decision

All immittance and audiometric results rule out any conductive hearing loss. The lack of an air-bone gap and the relatively poor speech recognition all fit with a diagnosis of sensorineural hearing loss. Note that the SRT is slightly poorer than the pure-tone average; this is observed in many elderly patients. Since there is nothing specific in the history to suggest a cause for the hearing loss, it is likely that the patient's advanced age is the etiologic factor. Improved understanding of slower speech, sometimes called "phonemic regression," is sometimes seen in patients with presbycusis. Convincing the patient to give hearing aids one more try will not be easy and should not be approached aggressively. This may come about if the patient feels a sense of confidence in you as an audiologist or if enrolled in coping strategies classes even without hearing aids.

HISTORY

Your patient is a 39-year-old female who complains of a sudden hearing loss following an automobile accident in which her car was struck from the rear. She also claims dizziness, severe bitemporal headaches, nausea, and "blackout spells." She did not mention tinnitus until asked about it during the history taking. There is no reported family history of hearing loss, ear infections, or other symptoms that the patient now claims to experience. She requests that a written report of your findings be sent to her for her "records."

DIAGNOSIS

Type of Loss Right: _____   Left: _____

Probable Etiology

_____

_____

Case Management

_____

_____

_____

_____

Reasons for Decision

_____

_____

_____

_____

AUDIOMETRIC DATA

Test	Right Ear	Left Ear
SRT	30 dB HL	35 dB HL
SRS	86%	80%
ARTs at 1000 Hz(ipsilateral)	85 dB HL	85 dB HL
ARTs (contralateral)	80 dB HL	85 dB HL
Static compliance	0.70 cc	0.73 cc
ABR	All waves normal; interpeak latencies normal; latency-intensity function normal	All waves normal; interpeak latencies normal; latency-intensity function normal
ABR Wave V threshold	15 dB NHL	20 dB NHL
TEOAE	Present	Present

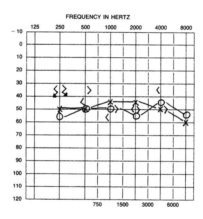

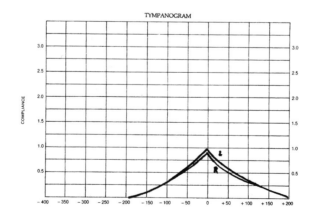

CORRECT DIAGNOSIS

Type of Loss

Right: Normal hearing
Left: Normal hearing

Probable Etiology

Nonorganic hearing loss (possible malingering)

Case Management

Complete as many tests for nonorganic hearing loss as time allows. Counsel the patient regarding her inconsistencies and accept the responsibility yourself for not having properly instructed her in taking the tests. Readminister the audiogram and SRT tests if time permits and arrange for rescheduling. Record all your findings in a report and file carefully. Do not confront the patient or act accusatory in any way. State in a separate report to her that inconsistencies preclude diagnosis and do not mention special tests for nonorganic hearing loss.

Reasons for Decision

The main indicator of nonorganicity in this case is the obvious discrepancy between the SRT and the pure-tone average for each ear (the former obtained at considerably lower hearing levels) and the normal acoustic reflexes. Normal ABR results and present TEOAEs suggest normal hearing in both ears. The history itself should have alerted you to possible nonorganicity since the patient may wish to bring suit for damages against the owner of the car that struck hers, but this is not evidence in itself. The primary behavioral tests for you to perform are pure-tone delayed auditory feedback and ascending-descending threshold exploration.

HISTORY

Your patient is a 7-year-old female who failed the public school hearing screenings on two occasions. The child's parents have had her examined by an otologist, who could find no explanation for the apparent high-frequency hearing loss and has referred her to you for further study. The child denies any difficulty in hearing.

DIAGNOSIS

Type of Loss Right: _____   Left: _____

Probable Etiology

_____

_____

Case Management

_____

_____

_____

_____

Reasons for Decision

_____

_____

_____

_____

AUDIOMETRIC DATA

Test	Right Ear	Left Ear
SRT	15 dB HL	20 dB HL
SRS	100%	100%
ART at 1000 Hz (ipsilateral)	90 dB HL	90 dB HL
ART at 4000 Hz (contralateral)	85 dB HL	95 dB HL
Static compliance	0.62 cc	0.59 cc
ABR	All waves normal; interpeak latencies normal; latency-intensity function normal	All waves normal; interpeak latencies normal; latency-intensity function normal
TEOAE	Present	Present

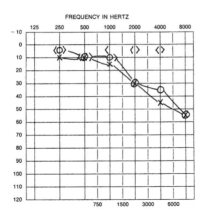

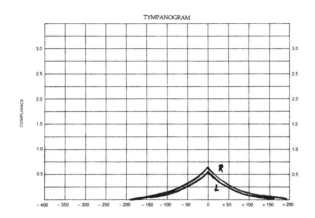

CORRECT DIAGNOSIS

Type of Loss

Right: Normal hearing
Left: Normal hearing

Probable Etiology

Collapsing ear canals

Case Management

Retest the child with insert receivers, stock earmolds, or plastic tubing in the ear canal to keep the canal open. If normal hearing is demonstrated, explain to the parents what has occurred and that failing the hearing test was no fault of the child. You may demonstrate to the parents how the canal collapses by placing an empty earphone cushion over the ear and allowing them to see the effect of ear canal closure through the opening. Send a letter to the referring physician with the correct audiogram and explanation of your findings.

Reasons for Decision

The high-frequency conductive hearing loss first seen in the absence of positive otological findings and the presence of normal tympanograms and acoustic reflexes are the main indications of collapsing ear canals. It is fairly easy to guess what happened in this case, but the same phenomenon can occur in the presence of a hearing loss, making diagnosis quite obscure. Careful examination at the time of otoscopy preceding immittance measures should alert you to possible collapsing canals. ABR and TEOAE results using insert earphones assist in the diagnosis of normal hearing but would probably not have been indicated in routine practice. This case gives testimony to the value of insert receivers. The supra-aural earphones used in the previous evaluation and in the previous school screenings created external ear canal collapse and false positive findings.

HISTORY

Your patient is a 16-year-old male who has had a hearing loss since early childhood when he became very ill with bacterial meningitis. He was educated in schools for deaf children using a manual approach, although he does have some speech. Use of amplification systems such as hearing aids and FM systems have consistently been unsuccessful. Recently his hearing was evaluated in the office of an otolaryngologist, who diagnosed a severe mixed hearing loss and recommended either exploratory middle-ear surgery (due to the air-bone gaps) or powerful hearing aids.

DIAGNOSIS

Type of Loss Right: _____   Left: _____

Probable Etiology

_____

_____

Case Management

_____

_____

_____

_____

Reasons for Decision

_____

_____

_____

_____

AUDIOMETRIC DATA

Test	Right Ear	Left Ear
SRT	NR	NR
WRS	Could not test	Could not test
ART at 1000 Hz (ipsilateral)	Absent	Absent
ART at 1000 Hz (contralateral)	Absent	Absent
Static compliance	0.60 cc	0.57 cc
ABR	NR	NR
TEOAE	Absent	Absent

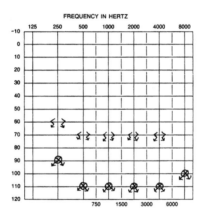

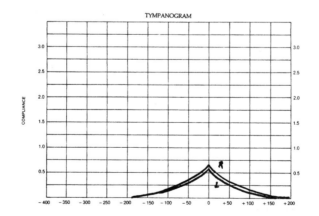

CORRECT DIAGNOSIS

Type of Loss

Right: Profound sensorineural hearing loss
Left: Profound sensorineural hearing loss

Probable Etiology

Severe cochlear damage due to childhood meningitis

Case Management

Retesting the patient with insert receivers instead of supra-aural phones results in no responses at the maximum limits of the audiometer. Moving the bone-conduction oscillator from the forehead to the mastoid process results in disappearance of the bone-conduction responses. These factors suggest that all the original responses were vibrotactile rather than auditory. Suggestion should be made to the physician that the apparent air-bone gap is false, obviating middle-ear surgery, and that the essentially total lack of response by air conduction makes successful use of hearing aids unlikely. The possibility of a cochlear implant may be pursued, as well as vibrotactile devices, but the family should be made aware of the limitations this may have considering the boy's systems of communication.

Reasons for Decision

The responses originally obtained near the limit of the audiometric equipment for air and bone conduction suggested the possibility of vibrotactile responses. The air-conduction responses disappeared with the use of insert receivers since they do not mechanically vibrate the skull to the extent that standard receivers do. The reason that the bone-conduction threshold became higher when the oscillator was moved to the mastoid was that tactile responses are known to require more intensity from the mastoid than from the forehead, and auditory responses require less intensity from the mastoid than from the forehead. Attempts at changing the patient's system of communication should be approached thoughtfully considering his history.

HISTORY

Your patient is a 79-year-old male, who has had a gradually progressive bilateral hearing loss for about fifteen years. He denies a history of ear infections or noise exposure. He experiences his greatest difficulties in discriminating speech in the presence of background noise. His main complaint is a sudden drooping of the right side of his face, which he attributes to a severe cold several days earlier. He says he thinks the paralysis may be "getting better." He states at the outset that he has no interest in purchasing hearing aids.

DIAGNOSIS

Type of Loss Right: _____   Left: _____

Probable Etiology

_____

_____

Case Management

_____

_____

_____

_____

Reasons for Decision

_____

_____

_____

_____

AUDIOMETRIC DATA

Test	Right Ear	Left Ear
SRT	15 dB HL	15 dB HL
SRS	88%	84%
ART at 4000 Hz (ipsilateral)	Absent	95 dB HL
ART at 4000 Hz (contralateral)	90 dB HL	Absent
Static compliance	0.50 cc	0.54 cc
ABR	All waves prolonged; interpeak latencies normal; latency-intensity function steep	All waves prolonged; interpeak latencies normal; latency-intensity function steep
TEOAE	Present	Present
Tone decay test at 4000 Hz	10 dB of decay in 60 seconds	15 dB of decay in 60 seconds

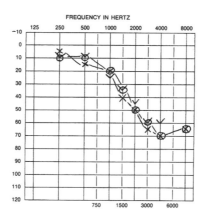

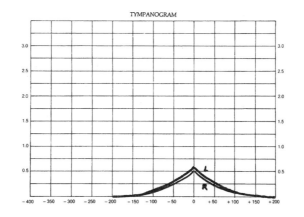

CORRECT DIAGNOSIS

Type of Loss

Right: Mild cochlear hearing loss
Left: Mild cochlear hearing loss

Probable Etiology

Presbycusis
VIIth cranial nerve damage (right); probably Bell's palsy

Case Management

Discuss the use of hearing aids without overstressing their potential value. Suggest that the patient see an otolaryngologist because of the facial palsy. Be as reassuring as possible without promising complete remission of the paralysis. Suggest retesting his hearing in one year, or sooner if he notices any change.

Reasons for Decision

The history and audiological findings are consistent with a cochlear lesion and, given the history, it is most likely produced by aging. The probability of Bell's palsy on the right side is suggested by the history of sudden onset, the trend toward spontaneous improvement, and because of the lack of ipsilateral and contralateral acoustic reflexes when the probe assembly of the immittance device is placed in the right ear (involving the right facial nerve). The facial paralysis is unrelated to the hearing loss.

HISTORY

Your patient is a 28-year-old female who complains of disturbing difficulties comprehending conversations within background noise. She states that she has trouble engaging in social interactions at parties, family gatherings, sporting events, and similar environments where noise levels are high. She reports that others seem to have little or no difficulty in these situations and that friends have begun to question her hearing abilities. In quieter listening environments she reports no difficulties. She has no history of ear infections, vertigo, or tinnitus and reports no current or past employment or recreational noise exposure. There is no reported history of hearing loss in her family. Given the history and the audiometric data on the following page make your diagnosis and substantiate it.

DIAGNOSIS

Type of Loss Right: _____ Left: _____

Probable Etiology

_____

_____

Case Management

_____

_____

_____

_____

Reasons for Decision

_____

_____

_____

_____

AUDIOMETRIC DATA

Test	Right Ear	Left Ear
SRT	0 dB HL	5 dB HL
SRS	96%	100%
ART (ipsilateral)	90 dB HL	95 dB HL
ART (contralateral)	90 dB HL	90 dB HL
Static compliance	0.35 cc	1.15 cc
ABR	All waves normal; interpeak latencies normal; latency-intensity function normal	All waves normal; interpeak latencies normal; latency-intensity function normal
TEAOE	Present	Present

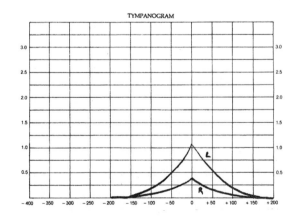

CORRECT DIAGNOSIS

Type of Loss

Right: Normal hearing
Left: Normal hearing

Probable Etiology

Obscure auditory dysfunction

Case Management

Discuss the normal test findings with the patient. Explain that while the underlying reason for her expressed difficulties is not always identifiable, that does not diminish the reality of the difficulties she is experiencing in social contexts. Having ruled out peripheral auditory dysfunction, outline possible underlying explanations for the difficulties, including anxiety or mild auditory processing problems surfacing only when listening conditions are more taxing. Offer to make referral for further evaluation of these possibilities if desired. Otherwise, in the absence of identifiable peripheral hearing disorder, treat the complaints as stemming from the basis of a situational hearing loss, providing counseling on communication strategies, employment of select assistive listening devices, and possible alterations in environmental/listening settings. Recommend a follow-up evaluation in one year, or sooner, if additional symptoms develop.

Reasons for Decision

The normal results for all tests rule out the presence of peripheral auditory pathology. The complaints presented by this patient are real and need to be addressed proactively in an effort to decrease their impact. Given the usual desire of patients to uncover etiology whenever possible, the discussion of potential etiologies and the offered referral for further evaluation is indicated.